CHINESE MEDICAL THERAPIES FOR DIABETES, INFERTILITY, SILICOSIS AND THE THEORETICAL BASIS

Edited by **Xing-Tai Li**

Chinese Medical Therapies for Diabetes, Infertility, Silicosis and the Theoretical Basis
http://dx.doi.org/10.5772/63167
Edited by Xing-Tai Li

Contributors
Wen-Long Hu, Jin-Wen Xu, Shuang Ling, Catherine Osgood, Guan-Cheng Sun, Ryan Lilly, Chi Chiu Wang, Shengjun Jiang, Xing-Tai Li

Published by InTech
Janeza Trdine 9, 51000 Rijeka, Croatia

Publishing Process Manager Dajana Pemac
Technical Editor SPi Global
Cover InTech Design team

First published February, 2017
Printed in Croatia

Additional hard copies can be obtained from orders@intechopen.com

Chinese Medical Therapies for Diabetes, Infertility, Silicosis and the Theoretical Basis, Edited by Xing-Tai Li
p. cm.
Print ISBN 978-953-51-2913-4
Online ISBN 978-953-51-2914-1

For EU product safety concerns:
IN TECH d.o.o., Prolaz Marije Krucifikse Kozulić 3, 51000 Rijeka, Croatia,
info@intechopen.com or visit our website at intechopen.com.

Meet the editor

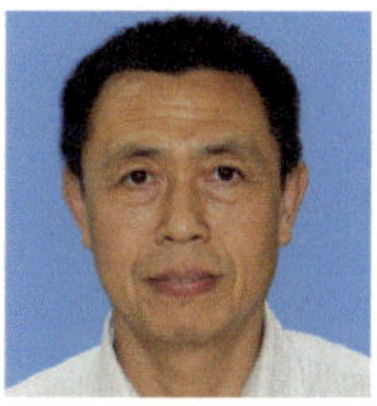

Xing-Tai Li was admitted to Peking University School of Pharmacy (pharmaceutics major) in 1996 and later transferred to Beijing University of Chinese Medicine, and from there, he received his PhD degree in basis of integrated Chinese and Western medicine-Biochemistry in 1999. He worked for 16 years as an associate professor in the College of Life Science, Dalian Nationalities University. His research interests include investigation on nature of Qi, the mechanism of Qi invigoration in TCM from mitochondrial bioenergetics perspective, and Qi-invigorating therapy for the prevention and treatment of mitochondrial diseases. He proposed a scientific hypothesis that Qi in TCM is bioenergy and demonstrated that the mechanism of Qi-invigorating action was implemented by improving mitochondrial energy metabolism.

Contents

Preface

Traditional Chinese medicine (TCM) is the summary of Chinese people's experiences in fighting diseases for thousands of years. Its theoretical system (Qi, Yin-Yang, five elements, etc.) is based on wisdom of ancient Chinese philosophy, embodies the Chinese people's own culture and profound speculative dialectical relationship between man and nature, and has made a great contribution to the health care of the Chinese people and the prosperity of the Chinese nation. TCM is the world's most comprehensive alternative and complementary medicine; its concepts and theories have been shrouded in mystery. With the advantages of Chinese medicines, including fewer side effects and greater effectiveness in some chronic complex diseases (such as infertility, cancer, and diabetes) than Western medicines, it was gradually accepted by foreigners and now has been spread to over 160 countries. In recent years, with the rising morbidity of serious illnesses like diabetes, infertility, silicosis, etc., there are no highly effective treatments; even though Western medicine has made spectacular advances, this influenced us to seek Chinese medical therapies of health care.

In the Chinese medical theories section, first chapter reviewed the effects of kidney essence (Jing)-, kidney-Yang-, kidney-Yin-, kidney-Qi-, and kidney-nourishing Chinese herbal formulas and single herbs on the kidney endocrine substances and proposed the idea that kidney endocrine substances are potential candidates of the material basis of kidney essence. Second chapter summarized in detail the Chinese medicines classified as contraindicated, not recommended, and cautiously used for pregnancy in Chinese Pharmacopeia. The authors obtained the most specific safety information for pregnancy and provided to the doctors, scholars, and patients a scientific evidence on the safe application of Chinese medicines during pregnancy. They gathered information about the adverse effects and potential toxicity of the Chinese medicines for pregnancy.

The major Chinese medical therapies are Qigong, herbal therapy, acupuncture, foods for healing, and Chinese psychology. In the Chinese medical therapies section, first chapter looked at how TCM views diabetes as well as new understandings of how Qigong can support the management of type 2 diabetes mellitus (T2DM). Second chapter reviewed the scientific evidence that kidney-nourishing Chinese herbal formulas, single Chinese herbs, acupuncture, and moxibustion are used for female and male infertility. Third chapter proposed a novel treatment method of silicosis by spraying with Chinese herbal Kombucha, which is made by fermenting extracts of herbs (tea, licorice, dried *Siraitia grosvenorii* fruit, and wild *Chrysanthemum*) with a Kombucha culture (containing two probiotics: *Gluconacetobacter xylinus* and yeasts).

Written for medical professionals, doctors, and readers interested in Chinese medicine, this book offers a unique perspective of Chinese medicine theories and therapies. It has practical chapters on diabetes, infertility, silicosis, kidney essence, and a compilation of contraindicated Chinese medicines for pregnancy. TCM is full of ancient Chinese wisdom and philosophical speculation and will provide new philosophical thinking and selective application for modern medicine. TCM is a treasure, and this ancient wisdom should be respected and applied to the modern medical system; it will provide more choices and a wider field of vision for Western medicine at the two cognitive crossroads of East and West.

Xing-Tai Li
College of Life Science, Dalian Nationalities University
Dalian, China

Section 1

Introduction

Introductory Chapter: Therapies Based on Kidney Essence and Qi in Chinese Medicine

Xing-Tai Li

Additional information is available at the end of the chapter

http://dx.doi.org/10.5772/67292

1. Introduction

Traditional Chinese medicine (TCM) is the precious treasure that Chinese nation accumulated in the process of struggling with disease for thousands of years, and she knows life and disease phenomenon in a unique perspective, is the important guarantee for the thriving of the Chinese nation, and is an immortal legend in the process of human civilization development. TCM is both a treasure trove of Chinese wisdom and the medical science based on ancient Chinese philosophy. TCM will provide new philosophical thinking and selective application for modern medicine. TCM theory on which it is based involves entities like Essence (Jing), Qi (Chi), and "meridians" that appear ambiguous, and the internal organs like the kidney and the spleen are understood very differently from those of modern anatomy. Even today TCM practitioners use these essential theories to understand, diagnose, and treat health problems.

2. The concept of "Essence" and "Qi"

"Essence" and "Qi," important categories in the ancient Chinese philosophy, are simple understanding of natural phenomena. The connotation and denotation of the concepts "Essence" and "Qi" are consistent in the ancient Chinese philosophy; both are invisible subtle materials existing in the universe with continuous movement and are the primitive composition of the universe, i.e., "Essence" is "Qi" and is also known as "Essence Qi." The concepts "Essence" and "Qi" in ancient Chinese philosophy were introduced into TCM, great changes about their connotation and denotation have taken place, and "Essence" and "Qi" became two concepts. "Essence" is the overall appellation on tangible materials inherited from the parents and acquired as useful subtle substances to the human body, is the most basic material that constitutes the Zang-Fu, tissues, and organs and maintains life activities of the human body, is the source of human life, and is also the origin of other life materials of the body.

"Qi" in TCM is the overall appellation on all the invisible subtle energetic materials in constant motion in the human body and functional activities of internal organs, is both an important part of the body, and is the power source of vital activities. In terms of its source, Qi originated from Essence and can be converted by Essence and is a more subtle material than Essence; Qi can also produce Essence, Essence, and Qi can be interconverted. In terms of its function, Qi can stimulate and promote the functional activities of the Zang-Fu organs and control the process of the human body; Qi is the fundamental that supports the life activity of the body, so when the movement of Qi stops, the end of life will arrive. Essence belongs to Yin, is tangible, and tends to be a material property; Qi belongs to Yang, is intangible, and tends to be a functional property. Essence is the material basis of viscera functional activities, and Qi is the motive force of promoting and regulating physiological activities of Zang-Fu organs.

Qi, as the master of the brain, regulates Yin-Yang and five elements, tonifies the five vital organs of the human body, keeps the six hollow viscera unobstructed, and is in charge of chemical and biological transformation and defenses. Qi of the human body comes from the congenital Essence inherited from parents, the refined food Essence transformed by the spleen, and the fresh air inhaled by the Lung. After birth, the congenital Essence is stored in the kidney to promote development and to control the reproductive activity of the human body. "Both life and death depend on Qi." Qi always underpins the basic theory of TCM and acts as its cornerstone. Qi has been used as a healing technique in China for 4000 years. This shows that Qi is closely related to health, disease, and life.

3. Qi and diseases

According to TCM, "Qi is the root of the human"; "All the diseases originate from Qi." Qi dominates the whole vital activities. Qi can make the human body work in an orderly fashion by promoting a variety of physiological activities; "Qi deficiency" will lead to a decline of physiological functions. As one part of a central medical classic *The Yellow Emperor's Inner Canon*, "Plain Questions" pointed out that consumption of the vital Essence Qi leads to deficiency. The basic idea of TCM to prevent and cure diseases is strengthening vital Qi to eliminate pathogenic factors. Strengthening vital Qi can improve body's resistance to disease, in order to eliminate weakness syndromes, ward off illnesses, and be physically strong. On the understanding of the etiology, TCM theory emphasizes the cause of disease—"vital Qi deficiency"—especially.

Xing-Tai Li proposes a scientific hypothesis that "Qi is bioenergy" [1] and Qi deficiency can lead to bioenergetic dysfunction, which can be improved by Qi invigoration and demonstrates that Qi invigoration was achieved through improved mitochondrial bioenergetics [2].

The central player in bioenergetics is the mitochondrion. Bioenergetic dysfunction is emerging as a cornerstone for understanding the pathophysiology of mitochondrial diseases. Mitochondrial dysfunction would undermine the function of cells, tissues, and organs, thereby causing cancer, diabetes, obesity, strokes, cardiovascular diseases, neurodegenerative diseases, aging, etc. Currently, there are no effective treatments, yet the causes of these diseases remain a mystery, while their incidence and morbidity either remain constant or are increasing. Huge investments in biomedical research in recent years have resulted in some striking accomplishments but have failed to reveal the anticipated causes for the diseases. Western medicine is in crisis [3]. According to TCM, Qi deficiency is the common cause of these diseases. Therefore, Qi-invigorating therapy can be used for mitochondrial diseases [4].

4. Kidney stores Essence theory

Essence Qi theory of ancient Chinese philosophy provides a premise condition to the birth of the Kidney stores Essence theory of TCM. Kidney stores Essence, Essence can be converted to Qi, and Qi converted by the Kidney Essence is Kidney Qi; therefore, if the Kidney Essence is sufficient, Kidney Qi is filling, and if the Kidney Essence is deficient, Kidney Qi fails. Kidney dominates growth, development, and reproduction of the body; this is the physiological function of Kidney Essence and Kidney Qi. Thus, the life processes of the human body, including birth, growth, prime, aging, and death, as well as reproductive ability, all depend on the rise and fall of Kidney Essence and Kidney Qi. Kidney Essence deficiency will result to insufficient reproductive Essence and ultimately lead to male infertility, female menopause, and infertility. Deficient Kidney Essence cannot produce enough Kidney Qi, so the sexual hypofunction will occur.

Kidney Qi can be divided into Kidney Yin and Kidney Yang, whose material basis is Kidney Qi, and they are the two different attributes of the Kidney Qi, of which Kidney Yin is the source of Yin Qi in the whole body and Kidney Yang is the root of Yang Qi in the whole body; the balance and coordination between Kidney Yin and Kidney Yang maintain the function of Kidney in TCM [5].

In Chapter 1, Shuang Ling et al. reviewed the effects of Kidney Essence-, Kidney Yang-, Kidney Yin-, Kidney Qi-, and kidney-nourishing Chinese herbal formulas and single herbs on the kidney endocrine substances and propose the idea that kidney endocrine substances, such as renin, kallikrein, erythropoietin (EPO), calcitriol, bone morphogenetic protein (BMP)-7, and klotho, are potential candidates of the material basis of Kidney Essence.

5. Kidney Essence, Qigong, and diabetes

Diabetes mellitus is a common degenerative disease and one of the leading causes of morbidity and mortality in developed countries. Diabetes has become a worldwide epidemic with a substantial social and economic burden [6]. The prevalence of this disorder is rising dramatically; an estimated 370 million people worldwide will be suffering from diabetes in 2030 [7]. Type 2 diabetes mellitus (T2DM) is a complex, chronic, metabolic disease with hyperglycemia and is the most common form of diabetes. The exact cause of T2DM is unknown in Western medicine. The modern studies show that bioenergetic dysfunction is emerging as a cornerstone for understanding T2DM. The mitochondria, whose main function is the production of the energy substance adenosine triphosphate (ATP), all the life activities depend on

ATP, mitochondrial dysfunction is at the centre of understanding many metabolic disorders, such as obesity and T2DM [8, 9]. Imbalanced energy homeostasis is characteristic of obese and T2DM patients [10]. This suggests that mitochondrial dysfunction might contribute to metabolic inflexibility and insulin resistance [11]. The ability of pancreatic β-cells to regulate blood glucose levels relies on mitochondrial ATP generation. Adenylate energy charge was decreased in prediabetic rats, as were ATP and adenosine diphosphate (ADP) levels. Conversely, adenosine monophosphate (AMP) levels were increased, evidencing a decreased ATP/AMP ratio [12].

Qigong is one of the major Chinese medical therapies used to strengthen Qi through self-practice and to manage the state of Qi to prevent and cure disease. Qigong therapies are popular in China as Qi therapies are in Asia. Medical Qigong is defined as the system of authentic Qi (vital energy) practice, which empowers the body to heal itself and to facilitate the healing process of others. Qigong exercises that focus on boosting Kidney and Spleen Qi can be particularly beneficial in managing T2DM [13–15].

Genetic, dietary, lifestyle, and environmental factors play a role in T2DM. Improper diet, overeating of certain foods, and overtaxing the body can weaken the Qi energy and disrupt the balance of the Zang (organs). Likewise, a sedentary lifestyle can weaken the Qi because not enough Qi is generated to invest in the strengthening of the body. Medical Qigong involves appropriate management and regulation of all energetic and informational communications. Receiving acupuncture treatments from an experienced Chinese medical practitioner supports the management of T2DM by improving the energetic function of the internal organs.

The kidney is central to the understanding of the pathogenesis of T2DM in Chinese medicine. Kidney is the root of Qi and the foundation of Yin and Yang in the body. The Kidney stores the Essence or one's inherited original reserves of vital energy. If one has constitutional kidney deficiency, one may already be deficient in Yin and may be predisposed to other organ imbalances. In the view of TCM, the etiology of diabetes can originate with pre-heaven Kidney Essence or Kidney Yin deficiency and weakness of the five Zang organs that predispose a person to further imbalances such as Spleen Qi deficiency. Congenital Kidney Essence and vital Qi deficiency are the intrinsic factors to diabetes. In addition, chronic Kidney Yin deficiency can diminish the generation of Kidney Yang. Combined Kidney Yin and Yang deficiency can in the long run lead to Kidney Qi failure, making the kidney unable to regulate the exiting of body fluids and manifesting as the need to urinate directly after drinking [16]. In Chapter 3, Guan-Cheng Sun et al. look at how TCM views diabetes as well as new understandings of how Qigong can support the management of T2DM and discuss the changes of mitochondrial energy metabolism and bioenergetics in the process of T2DM onset.

6. Kidney Essence and reproduction

Infertility is a worldwide problem affecting people of all communities; infertility has a wide range of causes stemming from three general sources: physiological dysfunctions, preventable causes, and unexplained issues [17]. It is an important medical and social problem in

http://dx.doi.org/10.5772/67292

the world as regards 15% of couples are infertile and 40% are infertile because of male factor infertility [18]. The ancient Chinese physicians think that the main pathogenesis of infertility is kidney deficiency; kidney-nourishing therapy is an effective method to the treatment of infertility. Kidney deficiency syndrome was positively correlated with Yin deficiency and Yang deficiency constitution. The Kidney stores Essence to control the reproductive activity. Kidney Essence is the basis of the conception; the Kidney Essence-, Kidney Qi-, Kidney Yin-, and Kidney Yang-tonifying therapies were often used according to treatment based on syndrome differentiation. Acupuncture and moxibustion work by regulating Qi flow over the meridians. According to the Yin and Yang theory, Kidney Essence pertains to Yin, while the Kidney Qi pertains to Yang. Kidney Essence is the most vital substance both constituting the human body and supporting its functional activities; it is the foundation of Kidney Yin and Kidney Yang. Kidney Yin provides material basis for the activities of human body, while Kidney Yang promotes the functions of the organs. In Chapter 4, Yen-Nung Liao et al. reviewed the scientific evidence that kidney-nourishing Chinese herbal formulas, single Chinese herbs, acupuncture, and moxibustion are used for female and male infertility.

TCM, with its long history of clinical practice, occupies an important place among the "alternative medicine" that has been gaining attention in recent years. Because of the general mildness in nature and the emphasis on relief, balance, and harmonization rather than forceful suppression, many good Chinese medicines are particularly suited for pregnancy. Lu Li et al. summarize in details the Chinese medicines classified as contraindicated, not recommended and cautiously used for pregnancy in Chinese *Pharmacopeia*. The authors obtained the most specific safety information for pregnancy. They gathered information about the adverse effects and potential toxicity of the Chinese medicines for pregnancy.

7. Silicosis and Qi deficiency

Silicosis is the most common pneumoconiosis globally, with higher prevalence and incidence in developing countries. To date, there is no effective treatment to halt or reverse the disease progression caused by silica-induced lung injury [19]. Effective therapies have to be found in order to reduce morbidity and mortality related to silicosis. In TCM, the lung dominates Qi of the body, the kidney is the root of Qi, and silicosis has close relations with the lung and kidney. The occurrence and development of silicosis are a chronic evolution process from the lung to the spleen and from the spleen to the kidney; finally, the lung, spleen, and kidney were all injured. Both Qi and Yin were injured, and vital Qi was depleted gradually. In Chapter 5, Shengjun Jiang et al. propose a novel treatment method of silicosis by spraying with Chinese herbal kombucha, which is made by fermenting extracts of Chinese herbs with a kombucha culture.

In summary, diabetes, infertility, and silicosis are either caused by or related to Kidney Essence and/or Qi deficiency in TCM, therefore, the introductory chapter subtitled "Therapies Based on Kidney Essence and Qi in Chinese Medicine." We hope you are interested in this book.

Author details

Xing-Tai Li

Address all correspondence to: xtli@dlnu.edu.cn

College of Life Science, Dalian Nationalities University, Dalian, China

References

[1] Li XT, Zhao J. An approach to the nature of Qi in TCM-Qi and bioenergy. In: Kuang H, editor. Recent Advances in Theories and Practice of Chinese Medicine. Rijeka: InTech Open Access Publisher, 2012. pp. 79–108.

[2] Li XT. Investigation on the mechanism of Qi-invigoration from a perspective of effects of Sijunzi decoction on mitochondrial energy metabolism. In: Sakagami H, editor. Alternative Medicine. Rijeka: InTech Open Access Publisher, 2012. pp. 247–275.

[3] Wallace DC. Mitochondria as chi. Genetics, 2008; 179(2): 727–735.

[4] Li XT, Kuang HX, Zhao J. Why is Qi-invigorating therapy in Chinese medicine suitable for mitochondrial diseases? A bioenergetic perspective. In: Saad M, editor. Complementary Therapies for the Body, Mind and Soul. Rijeka: InTech Open Access Publisher, 2015. pp. 243–283.

[5] Zhang L, Liu YY, Guo WX. Analysis of kidney Essence, Qi, Yin and Yang. Liaoning Journal of Traditional Chinese Medicine, 2013, 40(8): 1557–1560.

[6] Santos RX, Correia SC, Alves MG, et al. Mitochondrial quality control systems sustain brain mitochondrial bioenergetics in early stages of type 2 diabetes. Molecular and Cellular Biochemistry, 2014; 394(1–2): 13–22.

[7] Wild S, Roglic G, Green A, et al. Global prevalence of diabetes estimates for the year 2000 and projections for 2030. Diabetes Care, 2004; 27(5): 1047–1053.

[8] Gao AW, Cantó C, Houtkooper RH. Mitochondrial response to nutrient availability and its role in metabolic disease. EMBO Molecular Medicine, 2014; 6(5): 580–589.

[9] Andreux PA, Houtkooper RH, Auwerx J. Pharmacological approaches to restore mitochondrial function. Nature Reviews Drug Discovery, 2013; 12(6): 465–483.

[10] Corpeleijn E, Saris WHM, Blaak EE. Metabolic flexibility in the development of insulin resistance and type 2 diabetes: effects of lifestyle. Obesity Reviews, 2009; 10(2): 178–193.

[11] Galgani JE, Moro C, Ravussin E. Metabolic flexibility and insulin resistance. American Journal of Physiology-Endocrinology and Metabolism, 2008; 295(5): E1009–E1017.

[12] Rato L, Duarte AI, Tomás GD, et al. Pre-diabetes alters testicular PGC1-α/SIRT3 axis modulating mitochondrial bioenergetics and oxidative stress. Biochimica et Biophysica Acta (BBA)-Bioenergetics, 2014; 1837(3): 335–344.

http://dx.doi.org/10.5772/67292

[13] Sun GC, Zhou XH, Putiri AL, et al. Effects of Yi Ren medical Qigong on body weight in people with Type 2 diabetes mellitus: A secondary analysis of a randomized controlled pilot study. Journal of Integrative Medical Therapy. 2014; 1(1):1–5.

[14] Putiri AL, Lovejoy JC, Gillham S, et al. Psychological effects of Yi Ren Medical Qigong and progressive resistance training in adults with Type 2 diabetes mellitus: a randomized controlled pilot study. Alternative Therapies in Health and Medicine, 2012; 18(1): 30–34.

[15] Sun G. Cultivating the body's information system and experiencing the meridians through Qigong practice. The Journal of Traditional Eastern Health and Fitness, 2004; 14(1): 22–29.

[16] Cho CS, Yue KM, Leung WN. An outline of diabetes mellitus and its treatment by traditional Chinese medicine and acupuncture. Journal of Chinese Medicine. 2005; (78): 33–41.

[17] Amin U, Khan N, Bhat IA. Prevalence and causes of infertility among women of Jammu and Kashmir. International Journal of Development Research, 2015; 5(3): 3771–3774.

[18] Mahat R K, Arora M, Bhale DV, et al. Risk factors and causes of male infertility – A review. Biochemistry & Analytical Biochemistry, 2016; 5(2): 271.

[19] Lopespacheco M, Bandeira E, Morales MM. Cell-based therapy for silicosis. Stem Cell International, 2016; 2016(5): 1–9.

Section 2

Chinese Medical Theories

Chapter 2

The Connotation of Kidney Stores Essence Theory and Kidney Endocrine Substance

Shuang Ling, Yan-qi Dang, Rong-zhen Ni and
Jin-wen Xu

Additional information is available at the end of the chapter

http://dx.doi.org/10.5772/66972

Abstract

Traditional Chinese medicine (TCM) is a traditional healing system with unique theoretical system. The Zang-Fu theory is the closest mapping to body's physiological and pathological changes. Kidney is the most vital Zang organ in TCM system. However, the material basis of kidney essence is still undefined. In this chapter, we propose the idea that kidney endocrine substances, such as renin, kallikrein, erythropoietin (EPO), calcitriol, bone morphogenetic protein (BMP)-7, and klotho, are potential candidates of the material basis of kidney essence. In addition, kidney-nourishing therapy and related Chinese medicinal herbs are also introduced.

Keywords: TCM, kidney stores essence theory, renal endocrine, material basis, kidney nourishing therapy

1. Introduction

Traditional Chinese medicine (TCM) is one of the oldest medical treatments in the world. Limited by the times, it is characterized by the Yin-Yang, Five-Element, and Zang-Fu theory. The Zang-Fu theory explains the physiological function and pathological changes of human body, and the most vital organ would be the kidney. In western medicine, the kidneys are excretory organs with endocrine function. In TCM, it is not only related with anatomical concept but beyond of that. The material basis of kidney essence has long puzzled Chinese scientists. Dysfunction of hypothalamic-pituitary-adrenal (HPA) axis [1], hypothalamic-pituitary-gonadal (HPG) axis [2], and hypothalamic-pituitary-thyroid (HPT) axis [3] have been putting forward proposals. Nowadays, the stem cells self-control system depending on neuro-endocrine-immune (NEI) system regulated microenvironment [4] is the dominant academic view. Moreover, chromosome [5], vitamin D (calcitriol) [6], and erythropoietin (EPO) [7] were also considered to be the material basis of kidney essence. In modern medicine, the kidneys are endocrine organs that secrete a variety of hormones, such as renin [8], kallikreins [9], EPO [10], calcitriol [11], BMP-7 [12], and klotho [13]. This chapter aims to compare the similarities of the essence of kidney in TCM and the active substance secreting by the kidneys, and to propose the idea that renal endocrine function has the potential to be one of the kidney essence.

2. Kidney stores essence theory

2.1. Kidney stores essence (Jing)

Essence (Jing) is the basic substance both constituting the body and supporting its functional activities. The functions of essence are controlling reproduction, growth, and development, promoting the transformation of blood. For example, the forward movement of sperm in infertile men with kidney deficiency was much lower than that in fertile men, and the expression of c-kit mRNA, a marker of sperm damage, was increased [14]. For female, more than half of premature ovarian failure (POF) patients were differentially diagnosed by TCM as deficiency of kidney in 122 cases [15]. Destruction of the gonad was usually used to induce kidney deficiency animal model. Kidney-essence deficiency mice showed lower sperm density and motility, and lesser number of baby mice. The same is true for their descendants [16].

According to Suwen (Plain Questions), a classical work of the TCM theory, kidney essence controls the natural human processes from birth to death. There is an abundance of kidney essence in childhood, which provides the power to grow teeth, hair, and bones. During puberty, the kidney essence is even more plentiful resulting in the ability of fertility. Then female fertility begins to decline after 35 years old and male's after 40, as the kidney essence starts to decline. In old age, the kidney essence depletes as time passes, accompanying with infertility, osteoporosis, anemia, baldness, tinnitus, and even hearing loss. Therefore, aging is considered to be physiological kidney deficiency [17].

2.2. Kidney rules water

As urinary organs, TCM kidney and anatomical kidneys both bear consistency of functional. In the rat model of kidney-yang deficiency, classical kidney-nourishing formulas strongly regulated the RAA system hormone disorder [18].

2.3. Kidney governs reception of qi

According to the TCM theory, kidney controls deep and normal breathing in spite of the difficult-to-understand relationship between the kidneys and the lungs. It has been proved that kidney deficiency related closely with stable phase of chronic obstructive pulmonary disease (COPD) [19]. Geng et al. [20] found that the number of asthma attacks of children treated with tonifying qi and kidney TCM significantly decreased, and the effect remained after withdrawal of TCM for 9 months.

2.4. Kidney controls the bones

Stored in the kidneys, essence can transform into the marrow that fills up the bone cavities, where the blood is produced. The brain is even named as the "sea of marrow." For this reason, kidney essence is so important for bone development, healthy teeth, blood formation, and normal cognitive function. For example, the risk of fracture is significantly higher in chronic kidney disease (CKD) patients than in the general population [21]. The expenditures of oral problems also increased steadily along with the severity of CKD stages [22]. Homeostasis of calcium and phosphate maintain the development of bones. Many renal endocrines take part in the courses of bone metabolism, such as 1, $25(OH)_2D_3$, Klotho, BMP-7, and EPO. Aging may increase the risk of kidney dysfunction, and finally results in cardiovascular events, metabolic bone diseases, and even death [23].

When people are getting old, cognitive problems become more and more evident, such as amnesia, retard response, apathy, agnosia, and depression. The disorder of memory and cognitive deficit are usually related to Alzheimer's disease (AD) and vascular dementia (VD). TCM considered that the elderly person initially with kidney deficiency tends to have dementia. Promoting the transformation of blood is another function of kidney essence. Therapy of nourishing kidney [24] could promote the proliferation and differentiation of bone marrow hematopoietic progenitor cells *in vitro*.

2.5. The kidney influences the hair luster

Hair is nourished by the blood, which is generated from essence. Hairs collected from kidney deficiency patients [25] showed the shortest hair diameter and the relatively wide intervals between cuticles. Meanwhile, the levels of trace elements [26] and amino acids [27] in hair of patients with renal diseases decreased.

2.6. Ears as window of kidney

Presbycusis is regarded as a model of "kidney deficiency" deafness in TCM. The GC/MS analysis showed that hearing loss in the elderly people were positively correlated with kidney deficiency score in TCM [28]. It may be related to glutathione metabolism, amino acid metabolism, glucose metabolism, NMDA receptors, and GABA receptors. In addition, the ear length declined with the diminished kidney function after kidney donation [29].

In summary, the Five-Element theory serves to categorize all things in nature with the characteristics of five elements (**Figure 1**). Meridian tropism is used to explain the selectivity of drug action on a part of the body. For example, TCM considered that "salty flavor entering the kidney," "black food nourishing the kidney," and "correspondence of kidney with winter." Modern research has shown that salt is associated with the secretion of renin and the occurrence of high blood pressure. Black rice rich in several anthocyanins are effective in the prevention of hypertension [30].

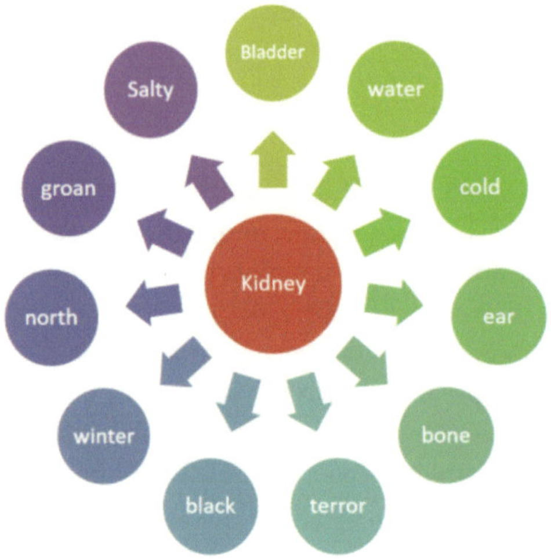

Figure 1. Categorization of kidney manifestation.

3. Renal endocrine and the "kidney stores essence" theory

According to the similarities of the kidney endocrine substances and the kidney essence in the sources and functions (**Figure 2**), we summarize several hormones secreted by the kidneys.

Renin is produced by renal juxtaglomerular epithelioid cells [8], and its secretion is with salt sensitivity [31]. Renin is believed as the regulators of kidney-yang, due to its participation in the blood pressure control system. In contrast, kallikrein-kinin system (KKS), mainly expressed in the distal tubules and collecting ducts of kidney [9], can lower blood pressure and promote the differentiation of stem cells, as the regulator of kidney-yin. Unlike the two above, EPO is exclusively secreted by renal interstitial fibroblast cells [10], which can regulate differentiation of red blood cells, stem cells, and progenitor cells. It is a veritable substance of nourishing blood. Calcitriol and BMP-7 are the presentations of the "kidney controls the bones" theory. The former is produced via 25-hydroxyvitamin D_3 1 alpha-hydroxylase (CYP27B1) in renal proximal tubular cells [11], while the latter is expressed in the renal outer medulla and in glomeruli, and in several glomerular cell types, such as mesangial, epithelial, and endothelial cells [12]. Knocking out BMP-7 in mice resulted in death shortly after delivery, with kidney failure, skeleton deformity, and eye loss [32].

As one of the material basis of the "kidney stores essence" theory, we will highlight α-klotho in this chapter. Klotho is mainly expressed in the distal tubule and the collecting duct [13]. As a longevity gene klotho has been widely known, as its reduction directly affects life expectancy [33]. Compared with the wild-type littermates, serum klotho level is reduced by approximately 80% in mice with renal-specific deletion of klotho, and exhibited severe growth retardation, kyphosis, and premature death. Serum α-klotho levels in healthy people rise with age to young adults and then gradually decline while age increased, showing a parabola [34]. The change of α-klotho level (**Figure 3**) is consistent with the description of kidney essence in Suwen.

http://dx.doi.org/10.5772/66972

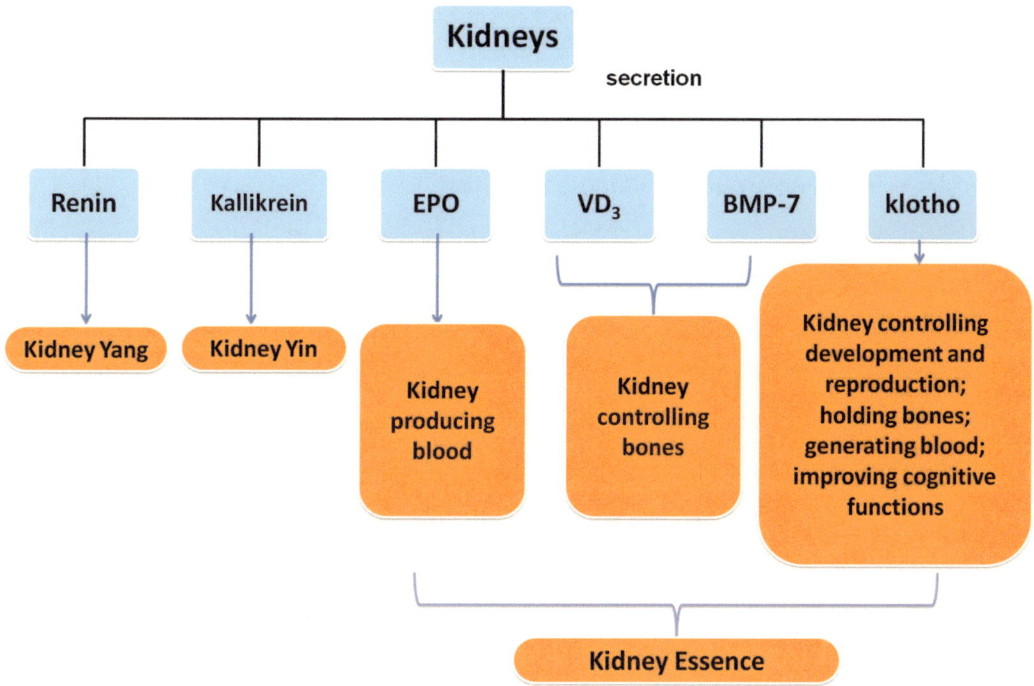

Figure 2. Similarity of kidney endocrine substances and kidney essence.

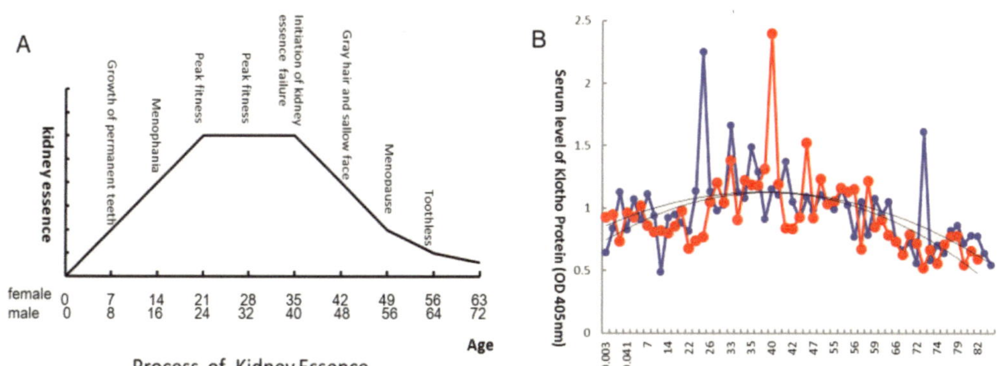

Figure 3. (A) Changes of kidney essence with age according to description of "Suwen." (B) Serum level of klotho protein changes with the human age [34].

Many studies have shown that α-klotho deficiency affects bone marrow stem cells and blood cell growth, development, and differentiation [35–37]. α-Klotho and EPO can be regulated by each other [38, 39]. Obviously, the role of α-klotho is very similar to the TCM theory of "kidneys essence generating marrow and producing blood."

Modern medical research has elucidated that α-klotho deficiency causes bone matrix protein distribution changes and calcification defect [40]; and participates in calcium and phosphorus metabolism [41]. α-Klotho also regulates the expression of vitamin D receptor [42]. It is clear that the lack of 1,25-dihydroxyvitamin D_3 can lead to osteoporosis [43]. Studies have shown that the introduction of variant KL-VS of the human KLOTHO gene in mice enhances cognitive function and increases serum α-klotho levels [44].

It has also been observed that there is a relationship between klotho and reproductive function [39]. The Nabeshima group also found that klotho-deficient mice have abnormal regulation of gonadotropins [45]. Recent studies have shown that maternal serum α-klotho exhibits positive association with fetal birth weight [46]. Our research shows that klotho expression in testis in 30-week-old SHR is significantly lower than that of normal controls Wistar-Kyoto (WKY) rats [47]. At present, although there is no direct evidence to prove the relationship between angiotensin II and klotho in testes, a lot of circumstantial evidence appears that klotho protect the organs and antagonistic effects of angiotensin II [48, 49]. Overall, we find that klotho function and the "kidney stores essence" theory have many overlapping and covering, reflecting the similarities between the two.

4. Reinforcing kidney drugs and diseases

There are many successful medical records of diseases treatment through kidney-nourishing therapy. For a good illustration of the fundamental role of tonifying kidney, as shown in **Table 1**, we summarize 10 common Chinese medical herbs for tonifying kidney and sum up their pharmacological activities.

2,3,5,4′-Tetrahydroxystilbene-2-*O*-β-D-glucoside (THSG) is the main composition of Polygonum Multiflorum (Thunb.) Harald., a traditional kidney-yin reinforcing herb. Our research has showed that THSG inhibited vascular aging [50] and regulated the expression of klotho, especially in the brain, testis, and kidney [47]. It also has the therapeutic benefits in bone diseases. For instance, THSG enhances the bone strength *in vivo* [47]. It has been reported that kidney-nourishing herbs improve the metabolism of calcium and phosphorus [51], regulate the levels of estrogen and 1,25-dihydroxyvitamin D_3 [52], and increase the activity of 1-α hydroxylase in renal disorder diseases [53]. Another kidney-yang nourishing herb, Epimedium brevicornu Maxim., and its active ingredient icariin can increase the klotho expression *in vitro* and *in vivo* [54]. The extract of polysaccharides of Cornus officinalis Sieb. et Zucc. [55] has a similar effect.

Bavachalcone, one of the effective components of Psoralea corylifolia L., is also a kidney-yang reinforcing herb. Our results demonstrated that bavachalcone not only prevents endothelial cells senescence [56, 57], but also promotes differentiation of bone marrow stem cells and endothelial progenitor cell via EPO/AMPK pathway (our unpublished data). Effects of kidney-nourishing herbs on differentiation of bone marrow mesenchymal stem cells also have been reported recently. For example, Epimedium brevicornu Maxim. enhances proliferation and osteogenic differentiation [58]; Davallia mariesii Moore ex Bak. stimulates differentiation into chondrocytes [59]; icariin facilitates differentiation into cardiomyocytes [60]; Rehmannia glutinosa polysaccharides

Chinese name	Latin name	Medicinal parts	Therapeutic efficacy
Yin-yang-huo (淫羊藿)	Epimedium brevicornu Maxim.	Whole-herb	To treat impotence and seminal emission, weak and cold and sterile, frequent urination and urinary incontinence, asthma, soreness and weakness of waist and knees, rheumatic arthralgia, hemiplegia, insensitivity of the limbs.
Bu-gu-zhi (补骨脂)	Psoralea corylifolia Linn	Dried fruit	To treat kidney-deficiency, backache, frequent urination, enuresis in children, leakage of protein or red blood cells in the urine, warming spleen and stopping diarrhea, asthma.
He-shou-wu (何首乌)	Polygonum multiflora (Thunb.) Harald.	Root	To treat light-headedness hemopenia, palpitation, insomnia, soreness and weakness of waist and knees, premature graying hair, tinnitus, spermatorrhea, constipation due to intestinal dryness, weakness by chronic malaria, rubella itching, carbuncle, scrofulous, hemorrhoids, hyperlipemia.
Tu-si-zi (菟丝子)	Cuscuta chinensis Lam.	Dried seed	To treat impotence and seminal emission, urine dripping after urination, frequent urination and urinary incontinence, soreness and weakness of waist and knees, eyes faint and tinnitus, threatened abortion, embryonic instability, diarrhea caused by deficiency of spleen and kidney, leukoderma.
Du-zhong (杜仲)	Eucommia ulmoides Oliver	Dried bark	To treat soreness and weakness of waist and knees, atrophy and weakness of foot and knee, dribble after voiding, genital damp itch, embryonic instability, threatened abortion, hypertension.
Shu-di-huang (熟地黄)	Rehmannia glutinosa	Prepared root	To treat liver and kidney Yin deficiency, soreness and weakness of waist and knees, osteopyrexia and fever, night sweat and spermatorrhea, blood-deficiency and pale complexion, palpitation, irregular menstruation, uterine bleeding and morbid leukorrhea, vertigo and tinnitus, premature graying hair, intrinsic heat and diabetes.
Gu-sui-bu (骨碎补)	Davallia mariesii Moore ex Bak.	Root and stem	To treat soreness and pain of waist and knees, vertigo and tinnitus, toothache and tooth mobility, injury and broken bones, alopecia areata, leukoderma.
Xian-mao (仙茅)	Curculigo orchioides Gaertn	Root	To treat impotence and cold semen caused by kidney-yang deficiency and yin-cold excess, urinary incontinence, abdominal cold-pain, soreness and pain of waist and knees, weak bones and lower limb spasm, menopausal syndrome.

Chinese name	Latin name	Medicinal parts	Therapeutic efficacy
Suo-yang (锁阳)	Cynomorium songaricum Rupr.	Succulent stem	To treat soreness and weakness of waist and knees, impotence and spermatorrhoea, constipation due to intestinal dryness.
Shan-zhu-yu (山茱萸)	Cornus officinalis Sieb. et Zucc.	Dried fruit	To treat soreness and pain of waist and knees, vertigo and tinnitus, impotence and spermatorrhoea, frequent urination and urinary incontinence, uterine bleeding and morbid leukorrhea, incessant sweating due to debility, intrinsic heat and diabetes.

Table 1. Ten kinds of kidney-nourishing herbs used in clinical treatments.

induces the formation of neuron-like cells or endothelial-like cells [61]; Curculigo orchioides Gaertn promotes differentiation into neurons [62]; and polysaccharides from Morinda officinalis How. and THSG promotes the proliferation and differentiation of bone marrow stem cells, and increases the number of peripheral blood cells in cancer chemotherapy [63].

Kidney-nourishing herbs also display effects of promoting cognitive function in type 1 diabetes and vascular cognitive impairment [64, 65]. Moreover, they successfully support the luteal insufficiency infertility [66]. Animal experiments further confirmed that the nourishing kidney treatment can promote ovulation and ovarian luteinizing hormone receptor expression in infertile rats [67].

5. Conclusion

Kidney essence declines with aging and leads to a variety of diseases, such as infertility, osteoporosis, senile dementia, aplastic anemia, and senility. Given the importance of kidney essence to life, researchers seek to understand the connotation of the "kidney stores essence" theory. Although "stem cells are congenital essence" is prevailing now, the plausible models and nonspecific indexes still need improvement. The kidney endocrine substances are similar with the kidney essence in their source and functions. It may have some help for the comprehension of the Zang-Fu theory and point to new targets for antiaging drugs. However, whether the kidney-nourishing medicine has implications on the kidney endocrine substance, still need further researching and discussing.

Author details

Shuang Ling, Yan-qi Dang, Rong-zhen Ni and Jin-wen Xu*

*Address all correspondence to: jinwen.xu88@gmail.com

Institute of Interdisciplinary Research Complex, Shanghai University of Traditional Chinese Medicine, Shanghai, China

References

[1] Zang-fu project team of Shanghai First Medical College. Disscussion on the entity of the kidney in TCM (Articles in Chinese). Chin J Internal Med. 1976; 1:80–85.

[2] Shen ZY, Wang WJ. Developments on kidney research in the view of integrative medicine (Articles in Chinese). J Integr Tradit W Med. 1988; 8(special II collection):8–10.

[3] Shen ZY. Shen (Kidney) of TCM on ancient and modern (Articles in Chinese). J Tradit Chin Med. 1997; 38(1):48–50.

[4] Zheng HX, Wang YJ, Li J, Lin SR. "Kidney Storing Essence" and dynamic balance between stem cell, microenvironment and NEI network (Articles in Chinese). Chin J Tradit Chin Med Pharm. 2012; 27(9):2267–2270.

[5] Zheng ML, Ruan SW. Hypothesis of the cell biology essence of Fivezang in TCM (II)—"kidney" and chromosome (Articles in Chinese). Chin J Basic Medi Tradit Chin Med Pharm. 2003; 9(11):60–63.

[6] Chen YZ, Qin Z, Wang YY, Guo J, Ma WD. Vitamin D as material basis of the kidney storing essence theory (Articles in Chinese). Global Tradit Chin Med. 2010; 03(6):447–448.

[7] Li YJ. Researches on EPO and nerve cells of YOU GUI YIN on kidney deficiency syndrome rats. Master Thesis, Southwest University. 2015.

[8] Celio MR, Inagami T. Renin in the human kidney. Immunohistochemical localization. Histochemistry. 1981; 72(1):1–10.

[9] Proud D, Knepper MA, Pisano JJ. Distribution of immunoreactive kallikrein along the rat nephron. Am J Physiol. 1983; 244(5):F510–F515.

[10] Maxwell PH, Osmond MK, Pugh CW, Heryet A, Nicholls LG, Tan CC, Doe BG, Ferguson DJ, Johnson MH, Ratcliffe PJ. Identification of the renal erythropoietin-producing cells using transgenic mice. Kidney Int. 1993; 44(5):1149–1162.

[11] Brunette MG, Chan M, Ferriere C, Roberts KD. Site of 1,25(OH)$_2$ vitamin D$_3$ synthesis in the kidney. Nature. 1978; 16; 276(5685):287–289.

[12] Kitten AM, Kreisberg JI, Olson MS. Expression of osteogenic protein-1 mRNA in cultured kidney cells. J Cell Physiol. 1999; 181(3):410–415.

[13] Hu MC, Shi M, Zhang J, Pastor J, Nakatani T, Lanske B, Razzaque MS, Rosenblatt KP, Baum MG, Kuro-o M, Moe OW. Klotho: a novel phosphaturic substance acting as an autocrine enzyme in the renal proximal tubule. FASEB J. 2010; 24(9):3438–3450.

[14] Zhang F, Liu JR, Ma YH, Ding CY, Yin HZ, Go SD. The value of SCF/c-kit in semen of infertile male with nephrasthenia syndrome (Articles in Chinese). J Hunan Univ Chin Med. 2016; 36(4):25–27.

[15] Teng XX. Syndrome analysis and Etiological Factor Survey of 122 patients with premature ovarian failure (Articles in Chinese). Chin J Inform Tradit Chin Med. 2008; 15(4):18–20.

[16] Sun J, Zhou AF, Zhou YY, Fang T. Kidney-jing deficiency reduces the fertility of male mice and their male offspring (Articles in Chinese). Natl J Androl. 2007; 13(8):754–757.

[17] Shen ZY, Huang JH, Lin W, Wang Q, Wu B, Liu XY, Zhang XM, Xu SX, Zhang WD. Transition of studying on kidney deficiency syndrome and aging from holistic concept to systematic biologic viewpoint (Articles in Chinese). Chin J Integr Tradit W Med. 2009; 29(6):548–550.

[18] Zhang S. The comparative research of different mechanisms of tonifying kidney between Kidney-qi Bolus and Yougui Bolus targeting at function of reproduction and RAA system (Articles in Chinese). Doctor Thesis, Shandon University of TCM. 2010.

[19] Chen HY, Hu XY, Zhou B, Xiong WZ, Hu L, Tan YL. Correlation analysis of pulmonary function in stable COPD classification and TCM syndrome type (Articles in Chinese). Hubei J Tradit Chin Med. 2012; 34(7):17–19.

[20] Geng Y, Wang W, Zhang J, Bi S, Li H, Lin M. Effects of traditional Chinese medicine herbs for tonifying Qi and kidney, and replenishing spleen on intermittent asthma in children aged 2 to 5 years old. J Tradit Chin Med. 2016; 36(1):32–38.

[21] Jamal SA, West SL, Miller PD. Fracture risk assessment in patients with chronic kidney disease. Osteoporos Int. 2012; 23(4):1191–1198.

[22] Huang R-Y, Lin Y-F, Kao S-Y, Shieh Y-S, Chen J-S. A retrospective case-control analysis of the outpatient expenditures for western medicine and dental treatment modalities in CKD patients in Taiwan. PLoS One. 2014; 9(2):e88418.

[23] Weir MR. Recognizing the link between chronic kidney disease and cardiovascular disease. Am J Manag Care. 2011; 17(Suppl 15):S396–S402.

[24] Tian C, Zhang XX, Zhang FF, Zhao ZJ, Cheng MX, Wang YC, Zhao J, Wu ZK. Effect of Bu-Shen Yi-Sui Sheng-Xue method for medicated serum of rats with aplastic anemia on mechanism of proliferation and differentiation of hematopoietic progenitor cells (Articles in Chinese). World Sci Tech Mod Tradit Chin Med. 2014; 16(5):1076–1082.

[25] Tang Q. SEM observation of scalp hair from people who deficiency of kidney-essence. Master Thesis, Hunan University of TCM. 2008.

[26] Sun DZ, Guo Z, Zhang JZ. The relation between hair trace elements and renal function. Acta Academic Med Neimongol. 2003; 25(1):27–29.

[27] Ba YM, Wang LQ, Yao J, Ding Z. Effect of Hushen No. II on hair growth characteristics and biomechanisms in patients with chronic kidney diseases at stage 1-4. J Guangzhou Univ Tradit Chin Med. 2016; 33(3):289–293.

[28] Dong Y, Ding Y, Liu PZ, Song HY, Zhao YP, Li M, Shi JR. Investigation of the material basis underlying the correlation between presbycusis and kidney deficiency in traditional Chinese medicine via GC/MS metabolomics. Evid Based Complement Alternat Med. 2013; 2013:762092.

[29] Katavetin P, Watanatorn S, Townamchai N, Avihingsanon Y, Praditpornsilpa K. Ear length and kidney function decline after kidney donation. Nephrology (Carlton). 2016; 21(11):975–978.

[30] Cassidy A, O'Reilly ÉJ, Kay C, Sampson L, Franz M, Forman JP, Curhan G, Rimm EB. Habitual intake of flavonoid subclasses and incident hypertension in adults. Am J Clin Nutr. 2011; 93(2):338–347.

[31] Hildebrandt DA, Irwin ED, Cates AW, Lohmeier TE. Regulation of renin secretion and arterial pressure during prolonged baroreflex activation: influence of salt intake. Hypertension. 2014; 64(3):604–609.

[32] Dudley AT, Lyons KM, Robertson EJ. A requirement for bone morphogenetic protein-7 during development of the mammalian kidney and eye. Genes Dev. 1995; 9(22):2795–2807.

[33] Kurosu H, Yamamoto M, Clark JD, Pastor JV, Nandi A, Gurnani P, McGuinness OP, Chikuda H, Yamaguchi M, Kawaguchi H, Shimomura I, Takayama Y, Herz J, Kahn CR, Rosenblatt KP, Kuro-o M. Suppression of aging in mice by the hormone Klotho. Science. 2005; 309(5742):1829–1833.

[34] Xiao NM, Zhang YM, Zheng Q, Gu J. Klotho is a serum factor related to human aging. Chin Med J (Engl). 2004; 117(5):742–747.

[35] Vadakke Madathil S, Coe LM, Casu C, Sitara D. Klotho deficiency disrupts hematopoietic stem cell development and erythropoiesis. Am J Pathol. 2014; 184(3):827–841.

[36] Sato S, Kawamata Y, Takahashi A, Imai Y, Hanyu A, Okuma A, Takasugi M, Yamakoshi K, Sorimachi H, Kanda H, Ishikawa Y, Sone S, Nishioka Y, Ohtani N, Hara E. Ablation of the p16(INK4a) tumour suppressor reverses ageing phenotypes of klotho mice. Nat Commun. 2015; 6:7035.

[37] Fan J, Sun Z. The antiaging gene klotho regulates proliferation and differentiation of adipose-derived stem cells. Stem Cells. 2016; 34(6):1615–1625.

[38] Hu MC, Shi M, Cho HJ, Zhang J, Pavlenco A, Liu S, Sidhu S, Huang LJ, Moe OW. The erythropoietin receptor is a downstream effector of Klotho-induced cytoprotection. Kidney Int. 2013; 84(3):468–481.

[39] Leone F, Lofaro D, Gigliotti P, Perri A, Vizza D, Toteda G, Lupinacci S, Armentano F, Papalia T, Bonofiglio R. Soluble Klotho levels in adult renal transplant recipients are modulated by recombinant human erythropoietin. J Nephrol. 2014; 27(5):577–585.

[40] Sasaki M, Hasegawa T, Yamada T, Hongo H, de Freitas PH, Suzuki R, Yamamoto T, Tabata C, Toyosawa S, Yamamoto T, Oda K, Li M, Inoue N, Amizuka N. Altered distribution of bone matrix proteins and defective bone mineralization in klotho-deficient mice. Bone. 2013; 57(1):206–219.

[41] Haussler MR, Whitfield GK, Kaneko I, Forster R, Saini R, Hsieh JC, Haussler CA, Jurutka PW. The role of vitamin D in the FGF23, klotho, and phosphate bone-kidney endocrine axis. Rev Endocr Metab Disord. 2012; 13(1):57–69.

[42] Forster RE, Jurutka PW, Hsieh JC, Haussler CA, Lowmiller CL, Kaneko I, Haussler MR, Kerr Whitfield G. Vitamin D receptor controls expression of the anti-aging klotho gene in mouse and human renal cells. Biochem Biophys Res Commun. 2011; 414(3):557–562.

[43] Peppone LJ, Hebl S, Purnell JQ, Reid ME, Rosier RN, Mustian KM, Palesh OG, Huston AJ, Ling MN, Morrow GR. The efficacy of calcitriol therapy in the management of bone loss and fractures: a qualitative review. Osteoporos Int. 2010; 21(7):1133–1149.

[44] Dubal DB, Yokoyama JS, Zhu L, Broestl L, Worden K, Wang D, Sturm VE, Kim D, Klein E, Yu GQ, Ho K, Eilertson KE, Yu L, Kuro-o M, De Jager PL, Coppola G, Small GW, Bennett DA, Kramer JH, Abraham CR, Miller BL, Mucke L. Life extension factor klotho enhances cognition. Cell Rep. 2014; 7(4):1065–1076.

[45] Toyama R, Fujimori T, Nabeshima Y, Itoh Y, Tsuji Y, Osamura RY, Nabeshima Y. Impaired regulation of gonadotropins leads to the atrophy of the female reproductive system in klotho-deficient mice. Endocrinology. 2006; 147(1):120–129.

[46] Miranda J, Romero R, Korzeniewski SJ, Schwartz AG, Chaemsaithong P, Stampalija T, Yeo L, Dong Z, Hassan SS, Chrousos GP, Gold P, Chaiworapongsa T. The anti-aging factor α-klotho during human pregnancy and its expression in pregnancies complicated by small-for-gestational-age neonates and/or preeclampsia. J Matern Fetal Neonatal Med. 2014; 27(5):449–457.

[47] Ling S, Duan J, Ni R, Xu JW. 2,3,5,4′-Tetrahydroxystilbene-2-*O*-β-D-glucoside promotes expression of the longevity gene klotho. Oxid Med Cell Longev. 2016, 2016:3128235.

[48] Zhou L, Mo H, Miao J, Zhou D, Tan RJ, Hou FF, Liu Y. Klotho ameliorates kidney injury and fibrosis and normalizes blood pressure by targeting the renin-angiotensin system. Am J Pathol. 2015; 185(12):3211–3223.

[49] Mitani H, Ishizaka N, Aizawa T, Ohno M, Usui S, Suzuki T, Amaki T, Mori I, Nakamura Y, Sato M, Nangaku M, Hirata Y, Nagai R. In vivo klotho gene transfer ameliorates angiotensin II-induced renal damage. Hypertension. 2002; 39(4):838–843.

[50] Han X, Ling S, Gan W, Sun L, Duan J, Xu JW. 2,3,5,4'-Tetrahydroxystilbene-2-O-β-D-glucoside ameliorates vascular senescence and improves blood flow involving a mechanism of p53 deacetylation. Atherosclerosis. 2012; 225(1):76–82.

[51] Yu S, Pei C, Dai L, Guo D. Effects of Bushen Jiangu Decoction on disorder of calcium and phosphorus metabolism and femoral bone mineral density in renal osteodystrophy rats (Articles in Chinese). Chin J Clin Healthcare. 2016; 19(01):78–81.

[52] Liu H, Li E, Tong X. Effects of replenishing Kidney herbs on estrogen and 1, 25- (OH) 2-D3 of dexamethasone-induced rats model with osteoporosis (Articles in Chinese). J Integr Tradit W Med. 1993; 13(9):544–545.

[53] Zhu F, Wang H, Gao L. Effects of kidney-nourishing herbs on renal 1-α-hydroxylase (Articles in Chinese). Shanghai J Tradit Chin Med. 2003; 37(12):42–44.

[54] Xinrong Z, Xiaoqin W, Changjiang W. Klotho gene expression in the remnant kidney model rats and the intervention effect of epimedium, astragalus and rhubarb compound (Articles in Chinese). Mil Med J S Chin. 2015; 29(3):196–199.

[55] Huihan F. Effect of polysaccharide from fructus corni on Klotho-Akt pathway and its downstream in hippocampus of the aged Wistar rats (Thesis in Chinese). Master Thesis, Jiamusi University. 2015.

[56] Dang Y, Ling S, Duan J, Ma J, Ni R, Xu JW. Bavachalcone-induced manganese superoxide dismutase expression through the AMP-activated protein kinase pathway in human endothelial cells. Pharmacology. 2015; 95(3–4):105–110.

[57] Dang Y, Ling S, Ma J, Ni R, Xu JW. Bavachalcone enhances RORα expression, controls small circadian transcription, and depresses cellular senescence in human endothelial cells. Evid Based Complement Alternat Med. 2015; 2015:920431.

[58] Li H, Li M, Li R, Wu L. Effects of epimedium on osteogenic differentiation of bone marrow mesenchymal stem cells. J Clin Rehabil Tis Eng Res. 2014; 18(6):979–984.

[59] Zhang H, Zhang Z, Xu H, Zhang X. Drynaria freeze-dried powder at different dosages influences proliferation and differentiation of rabbit bone marrow mesenchymal stem cells. J Clin Rehabil Tis Eng Res. 2014; 18(41):6649–6654.

[60] Wang Y, Wang H, Lv Y. Chinese medicine induces differentiation of bone marrow mesenchymal stem cells into cardiomyocytes. J Clin Rehabil Tis Eng Res. 2014; 18(1):155–160.

[61] Xiaopeng D. Supervisor: Hu Xiaomei. Effect of polysaccharides from plantago and rehmanniae on proliferation of bone marrow stem cells (Thesis in Chinese). Master Thesis, Chengdu University of TCM. 2009.

[62] Hi S, Lv W, Yang S. Chinese medical herbs Curculigo orchioides activates the directed differentiation from bone marrow stem cells into neuronal cells. J Chengdu Univ Tradit Chin Med. 2005; 28(4):8–11.

[63] Yan L. Supervisor: Xu Zhiwei. The study of tonifying the kidney to the regulatory mechanism of bone marrow stem cells in bone marrow suppression model (Thesis in Chinese). Doctor Thesis, Guangzhou University of Chinese Medicine. 2012.

[64] Ren Z, Luo W, Zhu L, Ho Y, Pan W, Chang X, Li X. Polygonum multiflorum downregulates MLCK expression in Type 1 diabetic rats and its effect on cognitive function (Articles in Chinese). Lishizhen Med Mater Med Res. 2015; 26(6):1314–1316.

[65] Feng J, Zang M. Clinical observation on treatment of mild to moderate vascular cognitive impairment with Liuwei dihuang pill (Articles in Chinese). Clin J Tradit Chin Med. 2010; 22(2):131–132.

[66] Zhong W. Treatment of luteal insufficiency infertility using based sequential therapy of nourishing kidney: a 48 caseses report (Articles in Chinese). Fujian J Tradit Chin Med. 2003; 34(4):16–17.

[67] Wang Y, Xiong Y. Effect of Bushen-Huayu Decoction on ovulation induction and ovarian luteinizing hormone receptor expression in infertile rats (Articles in Chinese). Chin J Tradit Chin Med Pharm. 2009; 24(5):656–658.

Chapter 3

Overview of Contraindicated Chinese Medicines for Pregnancy

Lu Li, Ling Shan Han, Xue Lu Jiang,
Ping Chung Leung and Chi Chiu Wang

Additional information is available at the end of the chapter

http://dx.doi.org/10.5772/67066

Abstract

Chinese medicines should be classified into drugs, which have both beneficial and harmful effects. For centuries, Chinese medicines have been widely used to relieve many symptoms and to treat complications during pregnancy. It is not clear how safe the Chinese medicines are being used during pregnancy and if there is any adverse effects to embryo-fetal development and prenatal and postnatal growth. Some Chinese medicines are indicated that they cannot be used in pregnancy. In this chapter, we will conduct a systematic review to summarize and characterize in details the Chinese medicines classified as contraindicated, not recommended and cautiously used for pregnancy in most updated version of Pharmacopeia of the People's Republic of China. Clinical reports including clinical trials, case reports, case series and animal studies including short-term and long-term toxicity, specific organ toxicity and different species of the Chinese medicines will be studied. Unlike those pharmaceutical drugs not recommend for use during pregnancy because of known or suspected adverse or teratogenic effects evident by animal studies and/or clinical trials, most of the Chinese medicines were utilized for long history in culture which, however, has very limited scientific data regarding the adverse pregnant outcomes.

Keywords: Chinese medicines, pregnancy, safety, review

1. Introduction

1.1. Chinese medicines for pregnancy

1.1.1. Application in China

Chinese medicines have become very popular and are widely applied to different kinds of medical conditions during pregnancy [1]. It promotes both mothers' and fetuses' health, relieves and cures common disorders in women [1]. It has been used as a main stream medicine in China with a longer history than Western medicines.

The first record of Chinese medicines treatment related to reproductive was first explained in A Chinese Bestiary 3000 years ago during Xia, Shang and Zhou era [2, 3]. Since then, Gu Rong was commonly used for contraception [2, 3]. In the following centuries, considerable progress was achieved in both clinical theory and practice while lots of milestones have been developed in Obstetrics and Gynecology. Due to historical factors of the late Qing Dynasty, and the influence of Western Medicine under the Renaissance, development of Chinese Medicine was less prominent [4]. After the establishment of People's Republic of China, with the great efforts of lots of Chinese Medicine practitioners and researchers, 6th edition of the textbook "Traditional Chinese Medicine in Obstetrics and Gynecology" [4] and lots of reference books and monographs have been published and used for daily teaching, training and self-learning. Apart from medical educations in Chinese Medicine, researches in collaborations with Chinese medicines and Western medicines have been raised to a new level and lots of meaningful conclusions have been drawn. For example, it was reported that combined Chinese medicines and Western medicines for ectopic pregnancy were more effective than conventional treatment [5, 6], and the method of combined medicines has been well studied and applied widely since then.

1.1.2. Development in foreign countries

Chinese Medicine in China has a long history, but its development for pregnant women in other countries is just within recent centuries. In foreign nations, the most common treatments are Acupuncture and Chinese herbal medicines (CHMs). Other therapies of Chinese Medicine, which could be used during pregnancy, began to spread to the world in very late twentieth century, such as Tui Na Massage and Die Da [4].

Chinese herbal medicines (CHMs) spread to the world earlier than acupuncture but only widely applied lately, due to the early advancement and modernization of Western medicines in foreign countries [7]. For instance, the "European Pharmacopoeia" had been locally well-developed, and Chinese herbs as medicines were not attractive to the practitioners and patients. With the advantages of Chinese medicines, including less side effects and greater effectiveness in some chronic diseases (such as infertility and irregular menstruation) than Western medicines, it was gradually accepted by foreigners and now has been spread to over 160 countries [3]. More and more foreign researchers and clinical doctors seriously have interests in it and come to China for further study.

1.1.3. Effectiveness and efficacy

With a long history of application of Chinese medicines to treat pregnant disorders, large amounts of case reports and clinical trials have been reported [8]. However, until now, limited data are available to overview Chinese medicines for pregnancy. Our team has reported in a systematic review [9] about the general applications, including common formulae, common individual CHMs, dosage and dosing, frequency, therapeutic efficacy, clinical indications and so on.

Chinese medicines are prescribed in formulae, and the Chinese medicine practitioners decide the formula according to the clinical presentation. Based on medical knowledge and personal experience, some use original or traditional formula, the others have individual prescription as personalized medicine. The prescribed formulae vary a lot, some formulae even lack unified theory and scientific evidence. Therefore, under a long-term collaboration with Cochrane Review Pregnancy and Childbirth Group, our team has conducted two systematic reviews with meta-analyses to study the claimed efficacy of Chinese herbal medicines for pregnancy-related disorders [10, 11]. The results showed that combined Chinese herbal medicines and other pharmaceuticals are more beneficial than other pharmaceuticals alone for threatened miscarriage [10] and unexplained recurrent miscarriage [11], but the evidence on the effectiveness and safety of Chinese herbal medicines alone as treatment is still insufficient, due to the poor qualities of the included clinical trials.

1.1.4. Safety

Safety is always the biggest issue in daily medical practice, and the issue is also a major concern to pregnant women. Chinese herbal medicines have been used to treat diseases and complications during pregnancy, and it is apparently well accepted as with fewer side effects.

There are 31 Chinese herbal medicines that were classified as toxic and contraindicated during pregnancy, which have been listed in many textbooks. The website of Chinese Medicine Council of Hong Kong (CMCHK) recently released another five CHMs, which contain aristolochic acid, which could induce abortion, kidney damage and cancer. Further studies of these Chinese herbal medicines have been carried out in the last 20 years and have demonstrated their adverse effects on both/either mothers and/or newborns. For example, Kansui Root (Radix Kansui, Gan Sui) is prohibited in pregnancy because it can poison the fetus and stimulate uterine contraction [12].

On the other hand, numbers of clinical trials have also been carried out to assess the safety of some Chinese herbal medicines in pregnancy and associated conditions, or to compare the adverse effects of Chinese herbal medicines with other medicines. Among the commonly used Chinese medicines, there are not too many studies of their potential harmful effects however. Our team has carried out a systematic review [13, 14] with meta-analyses to record the potential adverse effects and safety issues of CHMs as treatment for threatened miscarriage, but conclusive results remain elusive, as studies varied considerably in design, interventions and outcome measures. In the absence of placebo-controlled trials, the safety of Chinese medicines for the treatment of threatened miscarriage is unknown. Rigorous scientific and clinical studies to assess the possible risks of Chinese medicines are needed.

In conclusion, it is not clear how safe the Chinese medicines are being used during pregnancy and if there is any adverse effects to embryo-fetal development and prenatal and postnatal growth.

1.2. Chinese pharmacopeia

Unlike those pharmaceutical drugs not recommend for use during pregnancy because of known or suspected adverse or teratogenic effects evident by animal studies and/or clinical trials, most of the Chinese medicines were utilized for long history in culture which, however, has very limited scientific data regarding the adverse pregnant outcomes.

"Chinese Pharmacopeia", acknowledged by World Health Organization (WHO) as the official pharmacopeia for Chinese medicines, records 1146 different Chinese medicines [15]. It provides information on the herbs with their characteristics, identity, impurity, contents, extractum, analysis, property and channel, therapeutic action, pharmacological data, dose and dosing, precautious, storage, authentication methods and so on.

Among all this valuable information, we will obtain the most specific safety information for pregnancy from the Chinese Pharmacopeia and provide to the doctors, scholars and patients as scientific evidence on the safe application of Chinese medicines during pregnancy.

2. Objective

In this chapter, we will conduct a systematic review to summarize and characterize in details the Chinese medicines classified as contraindicated, not recommended and cautiously used for pregnancy in the most updated version of Chinese Pharmacopeia. Clinical reports including clinical trials, case series, case reports and animal studies including short-term and long-term toxicity, specific organ toxicity and different species of Chinese medicines will be studied.

3. Method

3.1. Search in Chinese pharmacopeia

Two review assessors carried out the word-by-word study in Chinese Pharmacopeia to identify the study medicines. First, they read all the recorded individual Chinese medicines and the formulae one by one and recorded in a list of the medicines remarked with application in pregnancy. Second, they checked the details of pharmaceutical effects and clinical functions and indications of these list-out medicines. If any adverse effects related to pregnancy were reported, the reference study would be traced and more details of the adverse outcomes were recorded, for further summaries and analyses. Third, they carried out the same rules to expand the search in different online databases, if the details of the adverse outcomes could not be accessed from the Chinese Pharmacopeia or the reference study. Finally, they extracted and summarized the specific safety information on three classifications of these Chinese medicines.

3.2. Search in other databases

To further supplement the pharmacological and toxicology data of the Chinese medicines, several online national and public resources on World Wide Web were also referred. It included Center for Food Safety and Applied Nutrition (CFSAN) from US Food and Drug Administration (FDA, (http://vm.cfsan.fda.gov/~dms/supplmnt.html), National Center

http://dx.doi.org/10.5772/67066

for Complementary and Alternative Medicine (NCCAM) from US National Institute of Health (NIH, http://nccam.nih.gov), Agricultural Research Service (ARS) from US Department of Agriculture (USDA, http://www.ars-grin.gov/duke), Medical Dictionary for Regulatory Activities (MedDRA) from International Federation of Pharmaceutical Manufacturers and Associations (IFPMA, http://www.meddramsso.com), National Council Against Health Fraud (NCAHF) from a private health agency (http://www.ncahf.org), Quackwatch from an American non-profit organization (http://www.quackwatch.com), HerbMed from Alternative Medicine Foundation (http://www.herbmed.org) and ConsumerLab from an independent laboratory (http://www.consumerlab.com), accessibility verified until 1 September 2016.

3.2.1. Search strategies for online databases

Search by subject heading/keyword/abstract/full text with:

1. Traditional Chinese medicines
2. Pregnancy
3. Western medicines
4. Comparisons studies
5. Safety
6. Toxicity

Or could be included or replaced by similar words:

1. Herbal medicines
2. Pharmaceuticals
3. Obstetric disorders
4. Pregnancy diseases
5. Therapy

Only clinical trials, which assessed the adverse pregnant outcomes of the Chinese medicines, were further selected for meta-analysis.

3.3. Study criteria

3.3.1. Types of studies

All published studies (list in Chinese Pharmacopeia and reference and reference of reference) that evaluated the safety of Chinese medicines for pregnancy were included. Studies of Chinese medicines for other clinical applications and in animal, chemical and basic research were included. (Non)/Randomized control trials, case controlled studies, case series, case reports, commentary articles and non-systematic reviews were excluded. Studies with no evaluation or incomplete records of adverse pregnancy outcome were also included.

Language of the publications was restricted to English and Chinese. Literature with either English or Chinese abstract should be available for initial search. No translation was required for Chinese articles as all review assessors can read Chinese and understand Traditional Chinese Medicine and Chinese medicines thoroughly. Translations were only sought from the language facilities of the university for articles written in English and Chinese.

3.3.2. *Types of participants*

There was no strict for types of participants, as we collected all safety information then further extracted for the summary table (**Table 1**).

3.3.3. *Types of interventions*

Since Chinese medicines are crude drugs of plant, animal and mineral origins, not only those Chinese medicines originated from plants or herbs but also those from animals and minerals were included. All types of Chinese medicine in either standard or combined formulas used during pregnancy or on pregnancy model animals regardless of the dose or duration of administration.

3.3.4. *Types of outcome measures*

General and specific adverse effects of the study Chinese medicines were recorded. Adverse reproductive outcomes in both mothers and fetuses/infants (both human and animals) will be recorded. Maternal outcomes included (1) toxicity (e.g. renal failure, liver failure, neurological impairment and death); (2) side-effects (e.g. anaphylaxis, gastrointestinal disturbance, hypertension/hypotension, cardiac arrhythmia, gestational diabetes and so on); (3) pregnancy loss (e.g. late abortion, intrauterine death and still birth) and (4) pregnancy complications (e.g. preterm/postdate labor, placenta previa, placenta abruption and so on). Fetal outcomes included (5) perinatal mortality (including prenatal and postnatal death); (6) toxicity (e.g. fetal compromise, neurological consequences, hydrops fetalis and so on); (7) congenital malformations and (8) neonatal complications (e.g. jaundice, infection, hypoglycemia and so on). Both long- and short-term adverse outcomes were reported and summarized.

3.3.5. *Data collection and analysis*

For each reference study to be involved in this review, all review assessors first screened the titles, abstract sections and keywords of every record to exclude the duplicates and obvious false positive. Second, full text of eligible studies was assessed for further inclusion or exclusion. If there was sufficient information and it met the inclusion criteria, the study was included in the analyses and summaries. Two review assessors assessed the studies for inclusion independently; any disagreement was resolved by discussion among all the review authors. The study authors were contacted for clarification if there were doubts about the eligibility of the study and the disagreement could not be resolved. The review authors were not blinded to the journal of origin or institution.

http://dx.doi.org/10.5772/67066

	CHM (English)	CHM (Biological name)	CHM (Chinese)	Dose	Actions and clinical indications	Classification in pregnancy
1	Aconiti kusnezoffii radix	Aconitum kusnezoffii Reichb.	草乌 (Cao Wu)	After preparation	To restore yang, to improve fire, and to disperse cold. Being used in: sweating profusely with body temperature dropping; muscle spasm in cholera; instant sweating, afraid of cold in cases of yangxu (yang deficient); pain and cold in chest and abdomen, chronic diarrhea due to pixu (spleen deficient), chronic muscle or joint pain due to wind cold dampness, tightness and pain in joints and muscles; edema and coldness in the lower legs due to shenyangxu (kidney yang deficient)	Contraindicated
2	Aconiti radix	Aconitum carmichaelii Debx.	川乌 (Chuan Wu)	After preparation	To restore yang, to improve fire, and to disperse cold. Being used in: sweating profusely with body temperature dropping; muscle spasm in cholera; instant sweating, afraid of cold in cases of yangxu (yang deficient); pain and cold in chest and abdomen, chronic diarrhea due to pixu (spleen deficient), chronic muscle or joint pain due to wind cold dampness, tightness and pain in joints and muscles; edema and coldness in the lower legs due to shenyangxu (kidney yang deficient)	Contraindicated
3	Anemones raddeanae rhizoma	Anemone raddeana Regel	两头尖 (Liang Toujian)	1–3	Rheumatism	Contraindicated
4	Aristolochiae fructus	Aristolochia debilis Sieb.et Zucc	马兜铃 (Ma Douling)	3–9	In coughs, phlegm, wheezing, blood in phlegm, with lung heat; hypertension, dizziness, with red face due to yinxu and liver yang ascending (gan yang ascending) condition; bleeding hemorrhoids and swelling in the anus	Contraindicated
5	Aristolochiae herba	Aristolochia debilis Sieb.et Zucc; Aristolochia contorta Bge.	天仙藤 (Tian Xianteng)	3–6	Same as 4	Contraindicated
6	Calomel	Calomelas	轻粉 (Qing Fen)	0.1–0.2	Use externally to kill parasites; for ringworms, boils and syphilis. Take internally to promote urination and bowel movements. Usually use with other water-removing herbs in difficulty in urination and defecation	Contraindicated
7	Cinnabaris	Mercury sulfide	朱砂 (Zhu Sha)	0.1–0.5	Insomnia	Contraindicated

	CHM (English)	CHM (Biological name)	CHM (Chinese)	Dose	Actions and clinical indications	Classification in pregnancy
8	Crotonis fructus	Croton tiglium L.	巴豆 (Ba Dou)	Proper dose	As laxative for constipation, distention, abdominal fullness and pain, caused by extreme coldness of bowels; for ascites; for clogged phlegm; for topical uses for abscesses and ulcers, to speed up ulceration of abscesses	Contraindicated
9	Crotonis semen pulveratum	Croton tiglium L.	巴豆霜 (Ba Doushaung)	0.1–0.3	Same as 8	Contraindicated
10	Curcumae rhizoma	Curcuma phaeocaulis Val.	莪术 (E Zhu)	6–9	Promotes qi flow and rids of blood stasis, amenorrhea due to blood stasis; distension and pain due to stagnation of undigested food; early stages of cancer in the cervix uteri (neck of uterus)	Contraindicated
11	Daturae flos	Datura metel L.	洋金花 (Yang Jinhua)	0.3–0.6	The flowers are being used in anesthesia, as sedative and for inducing sleep. The leaves are being used in rheumatoid arthritis. The seeds are being used in promoting blood circulation and in ridding of pain	Contraindicated
12	Erycibe schmidtii	Erycibe obtusifolia Benth.	丁公藤 (Ding Gongteng)	3–6	Rheumatism	Contraindicated
13	Euphorbiae pekinensis radix	Euphorbia pekinensis Rupr.	京大戟 (Jing Daji)	1.5–3	For edema, ascites, retention of phlegm, tuberculosis of lymph nodes. Can be taken internally or applied externally	Contraindicated
14	Euphorbiae semen	Euphorbia lathyris L.	千金子 (Qian Jinzi)	1–2	Dermatomycosis	Contraindicated
15	Euphorbiae semen pulveratum	Euphorbia lathyris L.	千金子霜 (Qian Jinzishaung)	0.5–1	Dermatomycosis	Contraindicated
16	Eupolyphaga steleophaga	Eupolyphaga sinensis Walker	土鳖虫 (Tu Biechong)	3–10	For blood stasis, amenorrhea, injuries of bones and muscles from impact, sprain in loin area	Contraindicated
17	Ferulae resina	Ferula sinkiangensis K.M. Shen; Ferula fukanensis K.M. Shen	阿魏 (A Wei)	1–1.5	Being used in ridding of parasites, improving meat digesting, treating purpura, epilepsy, enlarged liver	Contraindicated
18	Genkwa flos	Daphne genkwa Sieb. et Zucc.	芫花 (Yuan Hua)	1.5–3	For edema, ascites. For worm parasite: vinegar processed yuan hua, xiong huang. Make into powder. Take internally. For head fungal or ringworm: mix with lard and apply topically	Contraindicated

	CHM (English)	CHM (Biological name)	CHM (Chinese)	Dose	Actions and clinical indications	Classification in pregnancy
19	Gleditsiae fructus abnormalis	Gleditsia sinensis Lam.	猪牙皂 (Zhu Yazao)	1–1.5	Oral: for sequelae of strokes, losing consciousness, epilepsy with abundance of phlegm, difficulty in expelling phlegm, constipation. External usage: boils; breast engorgement in new mothers: wrap a peanut size powdered zhu ya zao in clean gauze. Dip it in 75% alcohol to wet the outer layer. Stuff it in the nostril (same side as the engorgement is) for 12 hours. If necessary repeat treatment after rested for 8 hours	Contraindicated
20	Ground beetle	Eupolyphaga sinensis Walker	䗪虫 (Zhe Chong)	3–10	For blood stasis, amenorrhea, injuries of bones and muscles from impact, sprain in loin area	Contraindicated
21	Hirudo	Hirudo nipponica Whitman	水蛭 (Shui Zhi)	1–3	For treatment of blood stasis, asthma, amenorrhea, physical injuries, unable to conceive, also used in abortion. Live shui zhi used externally in treating tumors, rid of swelling in boils, local blood clots (bruises)	Contraindicated
22	Hydrargyri oxydum rubrum	Hydrargyri Oxydum Rubrum	红粉 (Hong Fen)	Proper dose	Suppurative infection	Contraindicated
23	Hyoscyami semen	Hyoscyamus niger L.	天仙子 (Tian Xianzi)	0.06–0.6	Relieving spasm	Contraindicated
24	Kansui radix	Euphorbia kansui T.N. Liou ex T.P. Wang	甘遂 (Gan Sui)	0.5–1.5	Anti-inflammation	Contraindicated
25	Moschus	Moschus berezovskii Flerov	麝香 (She Xiang)	0.03–0.1	For coma due to stroke, angina, tumors and carbuncles, hastens delivery and facilitate the passage of stillborns. Seizures	Contraindicated
26	Mylabris	Mylabris phalerata Pallas	斑蝥 (Ban Mao)	0.03–0.06	For cancer, skin fungus infection, cancer of the lymphatic system, boils cannot ripen, dead tissues	Contraindicated
27	Nigellae semen	Nigella glandulifera Freyn et Sint.	黑种草子 (Hei Zhongcaozi)	2–6	For treatment of: heart palpitation, insomnia, weakness, cold or flu, cough	Contraindicated
28	Papaveris pericarpium	Papaver somniferum L.	罂粟壳 (Ying Suke)	3–6	Pain relief	Contraindicated
29	Pharbitidis semen	Pharbitis nil (L.) Choisy; Pharbitis purpurea (L.)Voigt	牵牛子 (Qian Niuzi)	3–6	Edema; ascites; constipation; difficulty in urination; beri beri; flatulence; abundance of phlegm, cough, asthma; abdomen pain with parasite	Contraindicated

	CHM (English)	CHM (Biological name)	CHM (Chinese)	Dose	Actions and clinical indications	Classification in pregnancy
30	Phytolaccae radix	Phytolacca acinosa Roxb.	商陆 (Shuang Lu)	3–9	Promote diuresis	Contraindicated
31	Realgar	Realgar	雄黄 (Xiong Huang)	0.05–0.1	Topical application for ridding of parasites: for scabies, ringworm, damp rashes, abscesses, ulcerations, snake bites. Taking internally for intestinal parasites, especially effective for roundworms. Dries dampness: expels phlegm	Contraindicated
32	Rhododendri mollis flos	Rhododendron molle G. Don	闹羊花 (Nao Yanghua)	0.6–1.5	Alleviates pain. Being used in rheumatoid arthritis, pain in broken bones, fungal infection of the skin	Contraindicated
33	Scolopendra	Scolopendra subspinipes mutilans L. Koch	蜈蚣 (Wu Gong)	3–5	Epilepsy, spasm, scrofula, sores, arthritis, hemorrhoid with pain, snake poison, scalding, leukemia, stroke	Contraindicated
34	Scorpio	Buthus martensii Karsch	全蝎(Quan Xie)	0.6–9	Epilepsy, stroke, paralysis, migraine, pain in arthritis, tetanus, tuberculosis in lymph nodes, urticaria, and bunacles	Contraindicated
35	Sparganii rhizoma	Sparganium stoloniferum Buch. -Ham.	三棱 (San Leng)	5–10	Painful menses. Postpartum complication, amenorrhea cause by qi stagnation and/or blood stasis. Cu san leng (prepared with vinegar) is stronger in pain inhibition. Fu san leng (stir fried with flour) is milder and is being used in promoting digestion	Contraindicated
36	Strychni semen	Strychnos nux-vomica L.	马钱子 (Ma Qianzi)	0.3–0.6	Rheumatoid arthritis, injuries, boils and swellings, sequelae from polio of children, impotence, for diseases of the gastrointestinal tract, organic and functional disorders of the heart and circulatory system, glycine encephalopathy, nervous conditions, myasthenia gravis; amyotrophic lateral sclerosis (als), cancer, depression, migraine, menopausal syndromes, facial neuralgias, raynaud's syndromes	Contraindicated
37	Strychni semen pulveratum	Strychnos nux-vomica L.	马钱子粉 (Ma Qianzifen)	0.3–0.7	Same as 36	Contraindicated
38	Toxicodendri resina	Toxicodendron vernicifluum (Stokes) F.A. Barkl	干漆 (Gan Qi)	2–5	Elimination of parasite	Contraindicated
39	Gleditsiae sinensis fructus	Moschus berezovskii Flerov	大皂角 (Da Zaojiao)	1–1.5	1. Dispels phlegm or coughs with abundance of phlegm; 2. Opens the orifices after strokes or epilepsies or facial paralysis due to excessive of phlegm; 3. Discharges puss when used externally for boils. Zao jiao ci uses: early stages of boils, difficulty in discharging of pus, eczema, and leprosy	Not recommended

http://dx.doi.org/10.5772/67066

	CHM (English)	CHM (Biological name)	CHM (Chinese)	Dose	Actions and clinical indications	Classification in pregnancy
40	Saussureae involucratae herba	Saussurea involucrata (Kar. et Kir.) Sch.-Bip.	天山雪莲 (Tian Shanxuelian)	3–6	For hardening of blood vessels of the brain, tumor. Folk applications include rheumatoid arthritis, impotence, irregular menses, placenta not being expelled after birth	Not recommended
41	Abelmoschi corolla	Abelmoschus manihot (L.) Medic.	黄蜀葵花 (Huang Shuhuaihua)	3–30	Promote diuresis	Cautiously used
42	Achyranthis bidentatae radix	Achyranthes bidentata BI.	牛膝 (Niu Xi)	5–12	Damp cold, weakness and pain in loin and knees, tight and spastic limbs, irregular menses, postpartum pain in abdomen due to blood stasis, afterbirth not being expelled, blood in urine, physical injuries and difficulty in bending knees. Raw huai niu xi is effective for breaking blood stasis. Cooked huai niu xi is effective for strengthening muscles and bones, promoting urination and strengthening essence of the body	Cautiously used
43	Aconiti kusnezoffii folium	Aconitum kusnezoffii Reichb.	草乌叶 (Cao Wuye)	1–1.2	Same as 1	Cautiously used
44	Aconiti kusnezoffii radix cocta	Aconitum kusnezoffii Reichb.	制草乌 (Zhi Caowu)	1.5–3	Same as 1	Cautiously used
45	Aconiti lateralis radix praeparata	Aconitum carmichaelii Debx.	附子 (Fu Zi)	3–15	Similar as 2	Cautiously used
46	Aconiti radix cocta	Aconitum carmichaelii Debx.	制川乌 (Zhi Chuanwu)	1.5–3	Same as 2	Cautiously used
47	Aloe	Aloe barbadensis Miller; Aloe ferox Miller	芦荟 (Lu Hui)	2–5	For constipation, dizziness, red eyes, and irritability due to heat buildup (yinxu (yin deficient) with heat). Kills intestinal parasites, especially roundworms. For treatment of ringworms. For burns and wounds. For treatment of liver yang over active	Cautiously used
48	Arisaematis rhizoma	Arisaeme erubescens (Wall.) Schott	天南星 (Tian Nanxing)	Proper dose	Being used in stroke with abundance of phlegm, paralysis, epilepsy, tetanus, tumors, arrhythmia. External use: insect and snake bites (grind with vinegar or water and apply to affected area)	Cautiously used

	CHM (English)	CHM (Biological name)	CHM (Chinese)	Dose	Actions and clinical indications	Classification in pregnancy
49	Arisaematis rhizoma preparatum	Arisaeme erubescens (Wall.) Schott	制天南星 (Zhi Tiannanxing)	3–9	Same as 48	Cautiously used
50	Aurantii fructus	Citrus aurantium L.	枳壳 (Zhi Qiao)	3–10	Indigestion due to low function; bloating in chest, abdomen and solar plexus area; constipation; diarrhea but difficult to expel, focal distention; fullness in the chest; cough with abundance of phlegm; prolapse of stomach, uterus and rectum	Cautiously used
51	Aurantii fructus immaturus	Citrus aurantium L.	枳实 (Zhi Shi)	3–10	Same as 50	Cautiously used
52	Borneolum	Cinnamomum camphora (L.) Presl	天然冰片 (Tian Ranbingpian) / 右旋龙脑 (You Xuanlongnao)	0.3–0.9	For fainting due to strokes or heat, bunacle, pain in joints, ulceration of the cornea, sores in the mouth, eczema, taking internally: mainly being used in pills; seldom in decoction. External application: for washing or added in external medication	Cautiously used
53	Borneolum syntheticum	Borneol	冰片 (Bing Pian)/ 合成龙脑 (He Chenglongnao)	0.15–0.3	Similar as 58	Cautiously used
54	Bovis calculus	Bos taurus domesticus Gmelin	牛黄 (Niu Huang)	0.15–0.35	Anti-inflammatory, anti-fever, anti-bacterial, opens the orifices, awakens the spirit, rid of phlegm. For high fever with delirium and convulsion due to hot diseases with hot phlegm, for chronic sore throat, for abscesses that have ripen and ruptured. Clears the heart, liver, relieves toxicity, rid of wind and tremors. For convulsions with high fever due to liver heat	Cautiously used
55	Bovis calculus artifactus	Bos taurus domesticus Gmelin	人工牛黄 (Ren Gongniuhuang)	0.15–0.35	Same as 54	Cautiously used
56	Bovis calculus sativus	Bos taurus domesticus Gmelin	体外培育牛黄 (Ti Waipeiyuniuhuang)	0.15–0.35	Same as 54	Cautiously used

	CHM (English)	CHM (Biological name)	CHM (Chinese)	Dose	Actions and clinical indications	Classification in pregnancy
57	Bufonis venenum	Bufo bufo gargarizans Cantor	蟾酥 (Chan Chu)	0.015–0.03	For food poisoning with stomach pain and bloating, vomiting with diarrhea, even fainting. Usually combine with she xiang, ding xiang, cang zhu, like formula called chan su wan. For bunacles, scofula, painful and swollen throat and various kinds of toothache: combine with xiong huang, ku fan, zhu sha, etc. Make into pills the sizes of mung beans. Take five pills each time with decoction of white portions of green onion. For scarlet fever usually combine with niu huang, xiong huang, bing pian, like liu shen wan. Being used in various types of cancer, like liver cancer, intestine cancer, leukemia, skin cancer, etc. Taking orally or external application has been successful to certain degree, according to some reports. Being used in respiratory and in circulatory exhaustion. It possesses the effect of raising blood pressure for long time. It also possesses respiratory stimulating effect	Cautiously used
58	Campsis flos	Campsis grandiflora (Thunb.) K. Schum.	凌霄花 (Ling Xiaohua)	5–9	Flower: for irregular menses, amenorrhea, tumors of the uterus, ovaries, endometriosis, mammary glands hyperplasia, chronic inflammation of the pelvic area, postpartum breast swelling, rubella, erysipelas, itchy skin, rosacea, acne. Roots: for rheumatoid arthritis, injuries from impact, broken bones, dislocations, acute infection of the digestive tract	Cautiously used
59	Carthami flos	Carthamus tinctorius L.	红花 (Hong Hua)	3–10	Actions and indications: 1. Being used in lumps in intestines and bowels, sores and carbuncles, pain from impact injuries, rheumatoid arthritis, invigorates circulation, breaks up blood stasis condition, and promotes menstruation: injuries from impact, swollen boils, irregular menses, pain in stopping of menses, pain from blood stasis after birth. Small amount can invigorate circulation and large amount can get rid of blood clots. It is an important herb in blood stasis therapy and often is prescribed with tao ren. To invigorate circulation, it is often used with dang gui, chuan xiong, shao yao. To rid of blood stasis, it is used with san leng, e zhu, and da huang; 2. Measles with blood stasis, color not lively red: use hong hua, dang gui, zi cao, da qing ye; 3. Angina of coronary diseases: use hong hua, dan shen, chuan xiong, chi shao; 4. Thromboangitis obliterans: use hong hua, dang gui, tao ren, chi shao, ru xiang; 5. For treatment of enlargement of the liver and spleen; 6. For physical injuries with blood stasis and pain: broken bones, dislocated joints, sprains, and impact	Cautiously used

	CHM (English)	CHM (Biological name)	CHM (Chinese)	Dose	Actions and clinical indications	Classification in pregnancy
****60	Cinnamomi cortex	Cinnamomum cassia Presl	肉桂 (Rui Gui)	1–5	Tonic for stomach, rid of wind, to promote sweating, for headache, anemia, cold limbs, to promote urination. To promote lung qi, in chill and fever, cold phlegm, diarrhea, muscle spasm, headache, back pain, sweating, to stop easily being annoyed, strengthening muscles and bones, promote circulation. Use in impotence due toshenyangxu (kidney yang deficient)	Cautiously used
61	Cinnamomi ramulus	Cinnamomum cassia Presl	桂枝 (Gui Zhi)	3–10	Same as 60	Cautiously used
62	Coicis semen	Coix lacryma-jobi L. var.ma-yuen (Roman.) Stapf	薏苡仁 (Yi Yiren)	9–30	For improving digestion, enhancing the lung function, ridding of bacterial or fungal infection, arresting pain and itchiness. For treatment of spastic muscles, arthritis pain in joints and muscular rigidity. Beri-beri and edema, vagina yeast infection, stones in the urinary tract, neualgia, difficulty in urination, lung abscess, gonorrhea, restless leg syndrome. Use raw yi yi ren for infection. Use stir fried yi yi ren for improving digestion	Cautiously used
63	Croci stigma	Crocus sativus L.	西红花 (Xi Honghua)	1–3	Similar as 59	Cautiously used
64	Cyathulae radix	Cyathula officinalis Kuan	川牛膝 (Chuan Niuxi)	5–10	Rheumatism, hematuria, amenorrhea, abdominal mass (fibroids of the uterus, ovarian cysts, endometriosis, pelvic inflammation, blood retention due to gynatresia, extra-uterine pregnancy, bleeding in the uterus, and other pelvic masses)	Cautiously used
65	Dianthi herba	Dianthus superbus L.	瞿麦 (Qu Mai)	9–15	Gonorrhea, edema, urinary tract inflammation, difficulty in urination, irregular menses, amenorrhea, dystocia, carbucle	Cautiously used
66	Dichroae radix	Dichroa febrifuga Lour.	常山 (Chang Shan)	5–9	Vomitting, malaria	Cautiously used
67	Echinopsis radix	Echinops latifolius Tausch.; Echinops grijisii Hance	禹州漏芦 (Yu Zhouloulu)	5–10	For boils, carbuncles, acute mastitis, unable to discharge milk	Cautiously used
68	Euphorbiae hirtae herba	Euphorbia hirta L.	飞扬草 (Fei Yangcao)	6–9	Relieve itching, lactogenesis	Cautiously used
69	Ferrous sulfate	Melanterite	绿矾 (Lv Fan)	0.8–1.6	Killing parasites	Cautiously used

http://dx.doi.org/10.5772/67066

	CHM (English)	CHM (Biological name)	CHM (Chinese)	Dose	Actions and clinical indications	Classification in pregnancy
70	Gendarussae herba	Gendarussa vulgaris Nees	小驳骨 (Xiao Bogu)	9–15	Furcture	Cautiously used
71	Haematitum	Haematitum	赭石 (Zhe Shi)	9–30	Liver yang over active, blurry vision and dizziness. Vomiting, hiccups, asthma; bleeding due to heat in the blood, excessive bleeding during menopause; chronic diarrhea; vagina yeast and bacterial infection; gastric neurosis	Cautiously used
72	I-borneolum/l-borneolum	Blumea balsamifera (L.) DC.	艾片 (Ai Pian)/ 左旋龙脑 (Zuo Xuanlongnao)	0.15–0.3	For fainting due to strokes or heat, bunacle, pain in joints, ulceration of the cornea, sores in the mouth, eczema, taking internally: mainly being used in pills; seldom in decoction. External application: for washing or added in external medication	Cautiously used
73	Impatientis semen	Impatiens balsamina L.	急性子 (Ji Xingzi)	3–5	Di gou cai (zhen zhu tou gu cao): rids of pain and dampness as in rheumatoid arthritis; invigorate blood, being used in rheumatoid arthritis, spastic muscles, eczema in the groin area, swollen boils, feng xian hua (feng xian tou gu cao): rids of pain and dampness as in rheumatoid arthritis, rid of toxin, being used in injuries, bruises, swelling, promoting menses, helping deliveries, expelling phlegm, tumors, snake and insect bites	Cautiously used
74	Leonuri herba	Leonurus japonicus Houtt.	益母草 (Yi Mucao)	9–40	As astringent, invigorate blood flow, promotes urination and rids of edema, rids of blood stasis, regulate menses, for premenstrual abdominal pain, infertility, post partum abdominal pain with lochioschesis (discharge in post delivery)	Cautiously used
75	Limonitum	Limonite	禹余粮 (Yu Yuliang)	9–15	Chronic diarrhea, bleeding not during menses, vagina discharge, hemorrhoids and hemorrhoids with bleeding or with pus	Cautiously used
76	Manis squama	Manis pentadactyla Linnaeus	穿山甲 (Chuan Shanjia)	5–10	Promote lactation, hastens boils to be ripen, expels pus, stop pain, pain in the joints of lower limbs, chronic malaria, rid of parasites. Unblocks menstruation, undo yu (blood stasis)., acute mastitis, ridding of wind dampness bi	Cautiously used
77	Melanteritum	Ferrous sulfate heptahydrate	皂矾 (Zao Fan)	0.8–1.6	Rid of toxins and dampness: being used externally on boils, skin ulcers, skin fungal infection. As tonic and rid of parasites: being used in edema due to deficiency; parasites and pain in the abdomen	Cautiously used

	CHM (English)	CHM (Biological name)	CHM (Chinese)	Dose	Actions and clinical indications	Classification in pregnancy
78	Meliae cortex	Melia toosendan Sieb. et Zucc.; Melia azedarach L.	苦楝皮 (Ku Lianpi)	3–6	Promote qi flow, rid of dampness-heat, clear liver fire, rid of pain, promote urination, regulates qi, kills parasites. Also used externally for fungus infections of scalp. Ku lian pi should be cooked longer than other herbs in the formula, because the active ingredients are more difficult to dissolve in water	Cautiously used
79	Momordicae semen	Momordica cochinchinensis (Lour.) Spreng.	木鳖子 (Mu Biezi)	0.9–1.2	Similar as 36	Cautiously used
80	Moutan cortex	Paeonia suffruticosa Andr.	牡丹皮 (Mu Danpi)	6–12	Clears heat and cools the blood, clears fire of yin deficiency, clear blood stasis and rid of clots, drain pus and reduces swelling due to blood stasis	Cautiously used
81	Myrrha	Commiphora myrrha Engl.; Commiphora molmol Engl.	没药 (Mo Yao)	3–5	For pain due to injuries, bruises, rheumatoid arthritis, tumors in the uterus, hemorrhoid, cataract, amenorrhea, bone and muscle ache, angina pectoris. External use on inflammation of the mouth cavity, periodontitis, wounds from cut not healing, and pharyngitis	Cautiously used
82	Natrii sulfas	Mirabilitum	芒硝 (Mang Xiao)	6–12	1. Constipation with dark urine, fullness and pain in abdomen; 2. Conjunctivitis; 3. Boils in mouth and tongue; 4. Swollen and painful throat area; 5. Tumor of the breast; 6. Stopping lactation; 7. Worm parasites of small children; 8. Red, swollen boils, before breakage	Cautiously used
83	Natrii sulfas exsiccatus	Natrii Sulfas Exsiccatus	玄明粉 (Xuan Mingfen)	3–9	Similar as 82	Cautiously used
84	Notoginseng radix et rhizoma	Radix Notoginseng	三七 (San Qi)	1–9	Raw san qi can stop bleeding and can transform blood stasis. It can stop bleeding without causing blood clots. It is widely used in injury medicine as in broken bones, swelling, impact injuries. Cooked san qi can be used as tonic	Cautiously used
85	Olibanum	Boswellia carterii Birdw.; Boswellia bhaw-dajiana Birdw.	乳香 (Ru Xiang)	3–5	Improves circulation, repairs muscle, as resolvent. Being used in: pain due to blood clots, spastic muscle, carbuncles, gum bleeding, gingivitis, rheumatoid arthritis, cirrhosis of liver, amenorrhea, physical injuries, ulcerated wounds not healing	Cautiously used
86	Persicae semen	Prunus persica (L.) Batsch	桃仁 (Tao Ren)	5–10	Breaks up blood stasis for constipation due to dry intestines for early stage of liver cirrhosis inhibits epstein-barr virus anti-tumor	Cautiously used

http://dx.doi.org/10.5772/67066

	CHM (English)	CHM (Biological name)	CHM (Chinese)	Dose	Actions and clinical indications	Classification in pregnancy
87	Physochlainae radix	Physochlaima infundibu-laris Kuang	华山参 (Hua Shanshen)	0.1–0.2	Relieve cough, resolving phlegm	Cautiously used
88	Polygoni cuspidati rhizoma et radix	Polygonum cuspidatum Sieb. et Zucc.	虎杖 (Hu Zhang)	9–15	For jaundice, gall bladder stones, blood stasis with menses stoppage, yeast infection, rheumatoid arthritis, physical injuries from impacts, inflammation of the bronchi, lobar pneumonia, poisonous snake bites, scalding injuries, acute hepatitis, urinary tract infection, boils, stoppage of menses due to heat in the blood, breast cancer, menopausal bleeding disorder	Cautiously used
89	Pruni semen	Prunus japonnica Thumb.	郁李仁 (Yu Liren)	6–10	Coprostasis	Cautiously used
90	Psammosilenes radix	Psammosilene tunicoides W.C. Wu et C.Y. Wu	金铁锁 (Jin Tiesuo)	0.1–0.3	Pain control	Cautiously used
91	Rhapontici radix	Rhaponticum uniflorum (L.) DC.	漏芦 (Lou Lu)	5–9	Similar as 67	Cautiously used
92	Rhei radix et rhizoma	Rheum palmatum L.	大黄 (Da Huang)	3–15	Lack of bowel movement, dysentery, blood clots, tumor, red and painful eyes, abdominal distention and/or pain, blood in stool, hemorrhoidal bleeding, urination burning sensation, nose bleeding, coughing up blood, sore extremities, edema, jaundice, lesions, burns and scalding (external application), absence of menses. Note: cooking for more than 10 minutes will reduce its purgative effect. For purgative effect use raw da huang. For blood invigorating action use wine or vinegar treated da huang. To stop bleeding use charred da huang	Cautiously used
93	Sappan lignum	Caesalpinia sappan L.	苏木 (Su Mu)	3–9	For vomiting, hiccups, burping, indigestion, and flatulence due to pixu (spleen deficient) or fungal infection; and for difficulty in expelling phlegm; chronic bronchitis; injuries from impact, dysentery, tetanus	Cautiously used

	CHM (English)	CHM (Biological name)	CHM (Chinese)	Dose	Actions and clinical indications	Classification in pregnancy
94	Selaginellae herba	Selaginella tamariscina (Beauv.) Spring	卷柏 (Juan Bai)	5–10	Improves circulation	Cautiously used
95	Sennae folium	Cassia angustifolia Vahl	蕃泻叶 (Fan Xieye)	2–6	Coprostasis	Cautiously used
96	Sulfur	Surphur	硫黄 (Liu Huang)	1.5–3	Coprostasis, killing parasite	Cautiously used
97	Tetrapanacis medulla	Tetrapanax papyrifer (Hook.) K. Koch	通草 (Tong Cao)	3–5	Being used in typhoid, paratyphoid with dark urine, pain in gonorrhea, edema scanty urine, and lack of mother's milk	Cautiously used
98	Trichosanthis radix	trichosanthes kirilowii Maxim.; trichosanthes rosthornii Harms	天花粉 (Tian Huafen)	10–15	Clears lung heat, dissolves phlegm, for cough with thick phlegm, rid of toxicity, expels pus; for treatment of chlorion epithelioma, hydatidiform mole	Cautiously used
99	Typhae pollen	Typha angustifolia L.	蒲黄 (Pu Huang)	5–10	Hei pu huang is pu huang that has been stir fried till dark color. It is being used in stopping bleeding. Raw pu huang possesses double effects of stopping bleeding and promoting circulation. For treatment of: angina: blood clot in the brain, high blood lipids, inflammation of the intestine and difficulty in urination: pu huang 50 g, xiong huang 10 g, bing pian 3 g, fresh white part of green onion 200 g,(wash the part of green onion and boil in water for 3 minutes. Smash all herb past it to the lower abdomen while still warm. Bleeding and abdomen ache due to chronic colitis: pu huang 3 g, wu ling zhi 3 g (wrap in cloth), baked ge gen 10 g, baked rou dou kou 3 g. Make into decoction and use as tea. External injury of the head with swelling: use raw pu huang and apply to the injury, 3 times a day. Bleeding in external injuries, hemorrhoids, boils, inflammation of the rib cartilage (without pus), rash in babies	Cautiously used
100	Typhonii rhizoma	Typhonium giganteum Engl.	白附子 (Bai Fuzi)	3–6	Similar as 2	Cautiously used
101	Vaccariae semen	vaccariae segetalis (Neck.) Garcke	王不留行 (Wang Buliuxing)	5–10	Promote diuresis	Cautiously used

http://dx.doi.org/10.5772/67066

	CHM (English)	CHM (Biological name)	CHM (Chinese)	Dose	Actions and clinical indications	Classification in pregnancy
102	Wenyujin rhizoma concisum	Curcuma wenyujin Y.H. Chen et C. Ling	片姜黄 (Pian Jianghuang)	3–9	Actions and indications: improves circulation of blood and qi, promotes flow of menses and relieves pain. For wind chill induced shoulder pain, mood fluctuations, schizophrenia, fever with dizziness, vomiting blood, nose bleeding, blood in urine, bleeding not during menses, jaundice, lower back pain, chest and abdomen pain caused by blood stasis, flatulence, pain during period of menses, injuries, bruises and swelling. Angina, treatment of pain in the rib area, gallbladder stones, postpartum pain. Today's application: high lipids, angina pectoris, rheumatoid arthritis, inflammation after surgery, periodontitis, tumor, acid dyspepsia, flatulent dyspepsia, atonic dyspepsia, shingles/herpes zoster, herpes simplex, coronary atherosclerosis, for inhibiting building up of b-amyloid, leukemia	Cautiously used

Similar: the clinical application and or the therapeutical effects of these CHMs are similar.

Same: (1) The CHMs are origin from different parts of a same plant or animal. (2) The CHMs are origin from the same part of the same plant or animal, but prepared in a different way for clinical medications.

Table 1. Summary of 105 CHMs for pregnancy [15, 16].

3.3.6. Data extraction, evaluation and management

Extraction form was designed and used to extract data. For eligible studies, two review authors extracted the data, any discrepancy was resolved through discussion or the third person was consulted. For each selected literature, publication year, study population, participant numbers, maternal age, gestation age, symptoms and signs, clinical diagnosis, examination and laboratory results, disease course, study intervention, standard or modified Chinese medicine formulas, individual medicine, immediate and follow-up outcomes were recorded. But only the data related to the safety classification and adverse outcomes would be reported in this review.

4. Results

4.1. Chinese pharmacopeia and literature study

There were 105 CHMs in Chinese pharmacopeia remarked with potential toxicity classification for pregnant women, of which 38 were "contraindicated", 2 were "not recommended" and 65 were "cautiously used" during pregnancy. Three of them were repeated under different common names, so we studied and collected information of 102 CHMs (**Table 1**) [15]. Some of the CHMs were origin from the same part of a plant, but they were prepared and applied in different format. Although their properties and safety outcomes were similar, we kept them separately list in the summary table.

An extension search on the cited references was carried out, and data of around another 600 studies were further extracted [15, 16]. A summary included the common name (English name), the biological name (Latin name), the original name (Chinese name), the recommended dose range in Chinese Pharmacopeia, clinical effects/indications and the safety classification in pregnancy of these 102 CHMs was reported in **Table 1**.

4.2. Adverse outcomes

4.2.1. General adverse effects and lethal effects

Among these 102 CHMs for pregnancy, around 80% were reported with their safety in clinical trials and or animal studies.

In those 38 "contraindicated" CHMs, 28 (73.7%) of which reported either general adverse effects or lethal effects (**Table 2**). About 16 of 38 (42.1%) CHMs were recorded with general adverse outcomes such as gastrointestinal discomfort including nausea, vomiting, lethargy, abdominal pain, diarrhea; nervous system problems such as drowsiness, headache, dizziness, respiratory failure, shock, dermatitis and ulcers, damage to multi-organ/systems, and so on. About 18 of 38 (47.4%) CHMs were recorded with lethal effects in human and mammals like mice, rats and rabbits. Immediate death was reported when Realgar Tragacanth (a component of Realgar) was orally administrated to mice, but details of the dose and dosing were not reported.

No.	CHM (English)	Adverse outcomes		Reproductive adverse outcomes	
		General adverse effects	Lethal effects	Maternal effects	Fetal effects
1	Aconiti kusnezoffii radix				
2	Aconiti radix		Death (human, po, 2–5 mg component)		
3	Anemones raddeanae rhizoma				
4	Aristolochiae fructus		Death (rabbit, ip, other details not available)	Stimulation on uterine muscle	
5	Aristolochiae herba				
6	Calomelas	Necrosis in multiple organs: heart, kidney, liver, lung, ovary (animals)			
7	Cinnabaris	Damage to heart, liver and kidney (mice, po, component 9.5 g/kg)		Decrease of pregnancy rate (mice, po)	
8	Crotonis fructus	1. Inducing dermatitis; 2. Sore throat, abdominal pain, watery diarrhea or bloody mucus, cyanosis, shock (human and animals)	Death (human, po, 20 drops)		
9	Crotonis semen pulveratum				
10	Curcumae rhizoma			Anti-pregnancy effect: interfere with implantation	Affect fetal growth
11	Daturae flos	Chromosome damage			
12	Erycibe schmidtii	1. Chronic toxicity on nervous system (mice); 2. Cardiac arrhythmias and death (rabbit, details not available)		Inhibition effects on uterus (pregnant rats)	
13	Euphorbiae pekinensis radix	Dermatitis	Death	Stimulation on pregnancy uterus	
14	Euphorbiae semen	1. Diarrhea; 2. Persistent abdominal pain, nausea, vomiting, lethargy, drowsiness (human)	Death (human)		

No.	CHM (English)	Adverse outcomes		Reproductive adverse outcomes	
		General adverse effects	Lethal effects	Maternal effects	Fetal effects
15	Euphorbiae semen pulveratum	1. Diarrhea; 2. Persistent abdominal pain, nausea, vomiting, lethargy, drowsiness (human)	Death (human)		
16	Eupolyphaga steleophaga				
17	Ferulae resina			1. Termination of pregnancy: induce miscarriage (pregnant mice, po, component 180 mg/kg); 2. Stimulation on pregnancy uterus (rabbit and mice)	
18	Genkwa flos			Termination of pregnancy: 1. Induce miscarriage (pregnant monkeys, amniotic injection for 1–3 days, component 0.2–8 mg); 2. Stimulation on pregnancy uterus (rabbit)	
19	Gleditsiae fructus abnormalis	1. Hemolysis; 2. Local mucosal irritation, damage to central nervous system, respiratory failure, death (mammals)	Death (mammals)		
20	Ground beetle				
21	Hirudo			1. Termination on pregnancy: 1.25 g/kg; 2. Termination on pregnancy: (ih on pregnancy d1, d6, d10, bid, decoction 2.5–3 g/kg)	
22	Hydrargyri oxydum rubrum		Death (component HgO_3)		
23	Hyoscyami semen	Chromosome damage			
24	Kansui radix	Hemolysis effect on quadriceps (rabbit)	Anti-fertility effects: placenta damage, miscarriage	1. Recorded embryotoxicity, but no malformation on fetus (rabbit, details not available); 2. Interfere with fetal circulation system	

No.	CHM (English)	Adverse outcomes		Reproductive adverse outcomes	
		General adverse effects	Lethal effects	Maternal effects	Fetal effects
25	Moschus		Death (mice, iv)	1. Stimulation on uterus, esp. Later stage of pregnancy (rabbit, puinea pig, rat); 2. Anti-early pregnancy and anti implantation	
26	Mylabris	1. Poisoning dogs and mice were liver and kidney damage (dogs and mice); 2. Acute poisoning of digestive, kidney, nervous system symptoms, such as blisters, ulcers, nausea and vomiting, oliguria, hematuria, dysuria, dizziness, blurred vision, high fever, shock and other symptoms (human, po)	Death (human, po, 3 g)		
27	Nigellae semen				
28	Papaveris pericarpium	1. Headache, dizziness, nausea and vomiting, constipation, urinary urgency and dysuria, sweating, biliary colic, the risk for respiratory depression; 2. Acute poisoning as lethargy, miosis, respiratory depression; 3. Infant poisoning can occur convulsions (human)			
29	Pharbitidis semen	Under large dose (animals): 1. Gastrointestinal irritation symptoms such as vomiting, abdominal pain, diarrhea, bloody mucus; 2. Kidney stimulation symptoms such as severe hematuria; 3. Nervous system such as language barrier, coma		Stimulation on pregnancy uterus (rat)	

No.	CHM (English)	Adverse outcomes		Reproductive adverse outcomes	
		General adverse effects	Lethal effects	Maternal effects	Fetal effects
30	Phytolaccae radix	Vomitting (cat, po, 2.5–10 g/kg), damage to brain (mice, po)			
31	Realgar		Immediate death (mice, po, component)		
32	Rhododendri mollis flos	Dermatitis	Death		
33	Scolopendra		Death (mice, intraperitoneal injection of high dose)		
34	Scorpio		Death (rabbit, iv, 0.5 mg/kg)	Specific toxicity: fetal malformation on bone developemnt	
35	Sparganii rhizoma		Death (mice, ip for 7 days)	Stimulation on uterus (pregnant rabbits)	
36	Strychni semen		1. Death (mice, details not available); 2. Death (human, po, 30 mg)		
37	Strychni semen pulveratum		1. Death (mice, details not available); 2. Death (human, po, 30 mg)		
38	Toxicodendri resina				
39	Gleditsiae sinensis fructus	Chronic toxicity (mammal, po)	Death (human, po)		
40	Saussureae involucratae herba				
41	Abelmoschi corolla				
42	Achyranthis bidentatae radix			1. Stimulation on non-pregnancy and early pregnancy uterus (mice); 2. Inhibition effects on both non-pregnancy and early pregnancy uterus (guinea pig); 3. Anti-fertility effect on pregnancy (mice)	
43	Aconiti kusnezoffii folium				
44	Aconiti kusnezoffii radix cocta				

No.	CHM (English)	Adverse outcomes		Reproductive adverse outcomes	
		General adverse effects	Lethal effects	Maternal effects	Fetal effects
45	Aconiti lateralis radix praeparata				
46	Aconiti radix cocta				
47	Aloe	1. local muscle necrosis (dog, muscle injection, high dose of decoction); 2. abdominal pain and pelvic congestion, nephritis.			
48	Arisaematis rhizoma	1. Weight loss, weakness, death, the water decoction of rabbit conjunctival irritation; 2. Emetic effect (mice, po, raw herb 40 g/kg)	Death (rabbit)		
49	Arisaematis rhizoma preparatum				
50	Aurantii fructus			1. Stimulation effects on uterus (rabbit); 2. Inhibition effects on uterus (mice)	
51	Aurantii fructus immaturus	Gastrointestinal expansion and salivate phenomenon (some animals, po)		1. Stimulation effects on uterus (rat and rabbit); 2. Inhibition effects on uterus (mice)	
52	Borneolum	1. Chronic toxicity to peripheral blood parameters and organ weight effects; 2. Liver damage (rat, po, 5 g/kg); 3. Neurotoxic effects (rat, po, 5 g/kg)		1. Induced abortion (mice, intraperitoneal injection once, 1/4,1/8,1/16ld50, either in early pregnancy (7–9d), mid pregnancy (10–14d) and late pregnancy (16–18d)) 2. Induction effect in mid and late pregnancy (mice)	
53	Borneolum syntheticum	1. Chronic toxicity to peripheral blood parameters and organ weight effects; 2. Liver damage (rat, po, 5 g/kg); 3. Neurotoxic effects (rat, po, 5 g/kg)		1. Induced abortion (mice, intraperitoneal injection once, 1/4,1/8,1/16ld50, either in early pregnancy (7–9d), mid pregnancy (10–14d) and late pregnancy (16–18d)) 2. Induction effect in mid and late pregnancy (mice)	

No.	CHM (English)	Adverse outcomes		Reproductive adverse outcomes	
		General adverse effects	Lethal effects	Maternal effects	Fetal effects
54	Bovis calculus	Fewer activities (mice, po, 7.5 g/kg)		Stimulation effects on pregnancy uterus and anesthesia uterus (rabbit, 0.9 mg component)	
55	Bovis calculus artifactus				
56	Bovis calculus sativus				
57	Bufonis venenum				
58	Campsis flos			1. Inhibition effects on mice non-pregnancy uterus (mice, 7.5 mg/ml); 2. Stimulation effects on pregnancy uterus	
59	Carthami flos	Low-spirited poisoning symptoms, reduced activity, walking difficulties (mice, intragastric and intraperitoneal injection, decoction)	Death (mice, intraperitoneal injection, component)	Stimulation effects on uterus (more obvious on pregnancy uterus than non-pregnancy one)	
60	Cinnamomi cortex				
61	Cinnamomi ramulus	The toxic effects of guizhi on mice have significant differences between day and night, the daytime toxic and lethal effects were significantly enhanced at night (mice)			
62	Coicis semen				
63	Croci stigma	Death (mammals)	Death (mammals)	Stimulation effects on both non pregnancy and pregnancy uterus (mice, puinea pig, rabbit, god, cat)	
64	Cyathulae radix			1. Stimulation effects on pregnant uterus (rabbit and cat); 2. Miscarriage rate 100% (mice, po for 7 days, component 2.5 g/kg)	
65	Dianthi herba			Stimulation on pregnancy uterine (rabbit and rat)	

No.	CHM (English)	Adverse outcomes		Reproductive adverse outcomes	
		General adverse effects	Lethal effects	Maternal effects	Fetal effects
66	Dichroae radix				
67	Echinopsis radix				
68	Euphorbiae hirtae herba			Increase miscarriage rate (pregnant mice, iv, 1.2 mg/kg on d8, d12 or d16)	
69	Ferrous sulfate	Vomiting, abdominal pain, diarrhea, dizziness and other adverse reactions			
70	Gendarussae herba				
71	Haematitum	Liver and lung damage (mice, po, 15–30% decoction)			
72	I-borneolum	1. Chronic toxicity to peripheral blood parameters and organ weight effects; 2. Liver damage (rat, po, 5 g/kg); 3. Neurotoxic effects (rat, po, 5 g/kg)		1. Induced abortion (mice, intraperitoneal injection once, 1/4,1/8,1/16ld50, either in early pregnancy (7–9d), mid pregnancy (10–14d) and late pregnancy (16–18d)); 2. Induction effect in mid and late pregnancy (mice)	
73	Impatientis semen			1. Anti-fertility effects (mice, po, decoction 3 g/kg); 2. Stimulation effects on uterus (mice, puinea pig and rabbit)	
74	Leonuri herba			1. Stimulation effects on uterus (mice, guinea pig, rabbit, dog, po, decoction and components); 2. Anti implantation and anti early pregnancy (mice, po, 0.1 ml for 4–5 times)	
75	Limonitum	Antifeedant, pulmonary congestion, hepatomegaly (mice, iv, decoction)			
76	Manis squama				
77	Melanteritum				
78	Meliae cortex	Stomach damage (rats) and inflammation (dogs)	Death (dogs, rabbits, monkeys, po, component)		
79	Momordicae semen				

No.	CHM (English)	Adverse outcomes		Reproductive adverse outcomes	
		General adverse effects	**Lethal effects**	**Maternal effects**	**Fetal effects**
80	Moutan cortex	Some central inhibition such as temperature decreasing, reflection disappeared, reduced activity, reduced respiratory, etc. (mice, intraperitoneal injection, component)			
81	Myrrha				
82	Natrii sulfas	Death (mice, intraperitoneal injection, decoction)	Death (mice, intraperitoneal injection, decoction)		
83	Natrii sulfas exsiccatus	Induce cancer			
84	Notoginseng radix et rhizoma	Acute and chronic toxicity reported, but details not avaliable			
85	Olibanum				
86	Persicae semen	Visible muscle relaxation, ataxia, piloerection and other phenomena (mice, intraperitoneal injection of 3.5 g/kg decoction)		Stimulation on pregnant uterine	
87	Physochlainae radix	Reduced activity, but recover on the next day (mice, intraperitoneal injection, 1 g/ml water extract)			
88	Polygoni cuspidati rhizoma et radix	Different degree of peritonitis, the severity and scope and dosage showed parallel effects, 700 mg/kg dose group was administered after 6 weeks can cause white blood cell count was significantly reduced, but there were no significant changes in blood and liver and kidney function. (rats, intraperitoneal injection, conponent)			

No.	CHM (English)	Adverse outcomes		Reproductive adverse outcomes	
		General adverse effects	Lethal effects	Maternal effects	Fetal effects
89	Pruni semen				
90	Psammosilenes radix				
91	Rhapontici radix				
92	Rhei radix et rhizoma	1. Long-term toxicity like cirrhosis and electrolyte metabolism (mice, po); 2. Overdose causes poisoning, nausea, vomiting, dizziness (mice, po).			
93	Sappan lignum				
94	Selaginellae herba				
95	Sennae folium				
96	Sulfur	1. Antifeedant and hepatomegaly (mice, po, decoction); 2. Overdose causes sulfur, central nervous damage and death (mice, po)	Death (mice, po, overdose)		
97	Tetrapanacis medulla				
98	Trichosanthis radix	1. Allergies (human, animals); 2. General toxicity: loss of appetite, damage to heart, liver and kidney, and central nervous system, death (female dog, im, 0.2–2 mg/kg)	Death (female dog, im, 0.2–2 mg/kg)	1. Miscarriage; 2. Stimulation effects on pregnant uterus (rabbit)	
99	Typhae pollen	1. Allergic reaction (guinea pig, intraperitoneal injection, decoction); 2. Hemolysis; 3. Reduction of red blood cells and white blood cells (mice)		1. Stimulation effects on uterus (mice, rat, puinea pig, rabbit) 2. Induction effects (puinea pig, mice, intraperitoneal injection, 50% dedcoction 3–2 g/kg) 3. Induced abortion (mice, po, decoction 10–20 g/kg)	Induced fetal death (mice, po, decoction 10–21 g/kg)
100	Typhonii rhizoma	Difficulty breathing, reduced activity, individual animal death (mice, po, decoction)	Individual animal death (mice, po, decoction)		

No.	CHM (English)	Adverse outcomes		Reproductive adverse outcomes	
		General adverse effects	Lethal effects	Maternal effects	Fetal effects
101	Vaccariae semen			1. Anti-implantation and decrease pregnancy rate; 2. Stimulation on pregnant uterus (rat)	
102	Wenyujin rhizoma concisum			1. Anti-fertility effects; 2. Anti-preganncy effects: termination of pregnancy; 3. Stimulation on uterus (mice, puinea pig, rabbit)	

Table 2. Adverse outcomes of CHMs for pregnancy [15, 16].

In 2 "not recommended for pregnancy" CHMs (**Table 2**), Gleditsiae Sinensis Fructus (Moschus berezovskii Flerov, DaJiaoZao) was recorded with both general effects of chronic toxicity in oral administration to mammals and lethal effects when human took a higher dose. No obvious adverse effects were recorded to the other CHM, Saussureae Involucratae Herba (Saussurea involucrata (Kar.et Kir.) Sch.-Bip., TianShanXueLian). Although it has great therapeutical function of improve the immune system, due to its pharmacological effects to enhance the blood circulation and stimulate the contraction of uterus, it may induce abortion during pregnancy, so it was not recommended for pregnant women.

In 65 "cautiously used" CHMs, 33 (50.8%) of which reported either general adverse effects or lethal effects (**Table 2**). About 24 of 65 (36.9%) CHMs were recorded with same general adverse outcomes such as gastrointestinal discomfort, nervous system problems, skin disorders and multi-organ damage. Other adverse effects such as muscle necrosis, pelvic congestion and cancer were also recorded. A total of 9 of 38 (13.8%) CHMs were recorded with lethal effects in human and mice. One study also reported that Meliae Cortex (Melia toosendan Sieb.et Zucc.; Melia azedarach L, KuJianPi) could cause death of rabbits, dogs and monkeys after oral administration of high dose of Toosendanin (a component), and the main reason is visceral bleeding, decreased blood pressure then acute circulatory failure.

4.2.2. Maternal and fetal adverse effects

Generally speaking, more maternal adverse effects were recorded than fetal effects. But this may be due to the failure of early pregnancy of mothers.

In those 38 "contraindicated" CHMs, 2 (5.3%) of which reported adverse effects on both mothers and fetuses (**Table 2**). A total of 12 of 38 (31.6%) CHMs were recorded with maternal adverse outcomes such as lower pregnancy rate (mainly due to anti-implantation), miscarriage (mainly due to effects on uterus), placenta damage and so on. About 3 of 38 (7.9%) CHMs were recorded with fetal adverse effects on bone development, circulation system and malformation.

No obvious maternal and fetal adverse effects were reported in those two "not recommended for pregnancy" CHMs (**Table 2**).

In those 65 "cautiously used" CHMs, 1 (1.5%) of which reported adverse effects on both mothers and fetuses (**Table 2**). About 20 of 65 (30.8%) CHMs were recorded with same maternal adverse outcomes as the "contraindicated" CHMs, and the study animals included mice, guinea pigs, rats and rabbits. Only 1 of 65 (1.5%) CHMs, Typhae Pollen (Typha angustifolia L, PuHuang), was recorded with mouse fetal death under oral administration of a 10–21 g/kg decoction.

4.3. Animal toxicity data

In **Table 3**, we summarized the toxicity data of those 102 CHMs from different animal studies and provided the information of LD50, dose, doing and species [15]. About 21 of 102 (20.6%) CHMs have more than one LD50 data, by applying raw herb, main/active components, water extraction and decoction or applying different species of animals. But 35 of 102 (34.3%) CHMs did not have a LD50 record. One implied reason is the CHM is too safe to test a LD50 data. Another reason is that half of these CHMs without a LD50 data were mineral origin, and there have been no study carried out to test their LD50 so far.

No.	CHM (English)	LD50	Dosing	Species	Remarks
1	Aconiti kusnezoffii radix	1.62–5780 mg/kg[4]	po, ip	Mouse	
2	Aconiti radix	0.3–18.0 mg/kg[1,4]	ig, iH	Mouse	
3	Anemones raddeanae rhizoma				
4	Aristolochiae fructus				
5	Aristolochiae herba	0.02 g/kg[1]	iv	Mouse	
6	Calomelas	410–2068 mg/kg[2]	ig	Mouse	
6	Calomelas	1740 mg/kg[2]	ig	Rat	
7	Cinnabaris	12.10 g/kg[2]	iv	Mouse	
8	Crotonis fructus	50–80 mg/kg[1]	iH	Rabbit	
8	Crotonis fructus	1 g/kg[1]	po	Rat	
8	Crotonis fructus	1600 mg/kg[4]	po	Mouse	
8	Crotonis fructus	600 mg/kg[1]	iH	Guinea pig	
9	Crotonis semen pulveratum				
10	Curcumae rhizoma	86.8 g/kg[1,4] raw herb	po	Mouse	
11	Daturae flos	8.2 mg/kg injection	iv	Mouse	
12	Erycibe schmidtii	6.22–8.85 mg/kg[1]	iH	Mouse	
13	Euphorbiae pekinensis radix				

No.	CHM (English)	LD50	Dosing	Species	Remarks
14	Euphorbiae semen				
15	Euphorbiae semen pulveratum				
16	Eupolyphaga steleophaga	146.45 mg/kg[1]	ip	Mouse	
17	Ferulae resina				
18	Genkwa flos	9.25 g/kg[2]	ip	Rat	
18	Genkwa flos	1.0–17.78 g/kg[1,2]	ip, ig	Mouse	
19	Gleditsiae fructus abnormalis				
20	Ground beetle	146.45 mg/kg[1]	ip	Mouse	
21	Hirudo	15.28 g/kg[2]	iH	Male mouse	Mouse, po, qd, decoction 500 and 1000 mg/kg, lower maternal weight, higher resorption rate, fetal malformation rate, higher neonatal mortality
22	Hydrargyri oxydum rubrum	22–120.98 mg/kg[1,2]	ig	Mouse	
22	Hydrargyri oxydum rubrum	18 mg/kg[1]	ig	Rat	0.1–1.5 g HgO_2 to human, death
23	Hyoscyami semen				
24	Kansui radix	30–346.1 mg/kg[1]	ip	Mouse	
25	Moschus	152–848 mg/kg[1]	ip, iv	Mouse	
26	Mylabris	1.71–1037 mg/kg[1,2]	ig, ip, iv	Mouse	
27	Nigellae semen				
28	Papaveris pericarpium	64–600 mg/kg[1]	iH, ip, po	Rat	
28	Papaveris pericarpium	20–745 mg/kg[1]	iH, ip, po, iv	Mouse	
28	Papaveris pericarpium	18–2200 mg/kg[1]	iH, iv, po	Rabbit	
28	Papaveris pericarpium	160–237 mg/kg[1]	po, ip	Guinea pig	
28	Papaveris pericarpium	MLD 60 mg/kg	iH	Cat	
29	Pharbitidis semen	37.5 mg/kg[1]	Ih	Mouse	
30	Phytolaccae radix	11.87–486 mg/kg[1,2]	ig, ip, iv	Mouse	
31	Realgar	3.207 g/kg	ig	Mouse	
32	Rhododendri mollis flos	0.25–5850 mg/kg[1,2]	ig, po, iv, ip, iH	Mouse	
33	Scolopendra	22.5–9900 mg/kg[1,2]	ig, ip	Mouse	

No.	CHM (English)	LD50	Dosing	Species	Remarks
34	Scorpio	2.4–10.3 g/kg[1,2]	iv, ip	Mouse	
35	Sparganii rhizoma	55.8–233.3 g/kg[3] raw herb	ip	Mouse	
36	Strychni semen	1.53–301.9 mg/kg[1,2,4]	ig, ip	Mouse	
37	Strychni semen pulveratum	301.9 mg/kg[2]	ig	Mouse	
38	Toxicodendri resina				
39	Gleditsiae sinensis fructus				
40	Saussureae involucratae herba				
41	Abelmoschi corolla				
42	Achyranthis bidentatae radix	6.4–146.49 g/kg[1]	ig, ip	Mouse	
43	Aconiti kusnezoffii folium				
44	Aconiti kusnezoffii radix cocta				
45	Aconiti lateralis radix praeparata	0.1–17400 mg/kg[1,2]	ig, iv, ip, Ih	Mouse	
45	Aconiti lateralis radix praeparata	0.102 mg/kg (minimum lethal dose)	iv	Rat	
45	Aconiti lateralis radix praeparata	0.075–1.65 mg/kg[1]	iv	Frog	
45	Aconiti lateralis radix praeparata	0.04–0.05 mg/kg[1]	iv	Rabbit	
45	Aconiti lateralis radix praeparata	0.06–0.12 mg/kg[1]	iv	Guinea pig	
46	Aconiti radix cocta				
47	Aloe				
48	Arisaematis rhizoma	13.5–210 g/kg[1,2,4]	ig, ip	Mouse	
49	Arisaematis rhizoma preparatum				
50	Aurantii fructus				
51	Aurantii fructus immaturus	71.8–267 g/kg[2]	iv, ip	Mouse	
52	Borneolum	907–4960 mg/kg[1]	ig, ip	Mouse	

No.	CHM (English)	LD50	Dosing	Species	Remarks
53	Borneolum syntheticum	907–4960 mg/kg[1]	ig, ip	Mouse	
54	Bovis calculus	497.5–6630 mg/kg[1]	ig, ip, iv	Mouse	
55	Bovis calculus artifactus				
56	Bovis calculus sativus				
57	Bufonis venenum				
58	Campsis flos	50 g/kg (raw herb, maximum tolerated dose)	ig	Mouse	
59	Carthami flos	2.35–20.7 g/kg[1,2]	ig, ig, iv	Mouse	
60	Cinnamomi cortex	42–46 g/kg[1,2]	ip	Mouse	
61	Cinnamomi ramulus	624.7(daytime)–773.6(night)mg/kg[2]	ig	Mouse	
62	Coicis semen	10 ml/kg[1] (maximum tolerated dose)	po	Mouse	
63	Croci stigma	20.7 g/kg[1]	po	Mouse	
64	Cyathulae radix				
65	Dianthi herba				
66	Dichroae radix				
67	Echinopsis radix				
68	Euphorbiae hirtae herba				
69	Ferrous sulfate				
70	Gendarussae herba				
71	Haematitum	12.90 g/kg[2]	iv	Mouse	
72	I-borneolum	907–4960 mg/kg[1]	ig, ip	Mouse	
73	Impatientis semen				
74	Leonuri herba	0.572–60 g/kg[1,2]	iv	Mouse	
75	Limonitum	8.25 g/kg[2]	iv	Mouse	
76	Manis squama				
77	Melanteritum				
78	Meliae cortex	13.8–244.2 mg/kg[1]	ip, iv, iH, po	Mouse	
78	Meliae cortex	9.8 mg/kg[1]	iH	Rat	
78	Meliae cortex	4.2 mg/kg[1]	iv	Rabbit	
79	Momordicae semen				

No.	CHM (English)	LD50	Dosing	Species	Remarks
80	Moutan cortex	196–6900 mg/kg[1]	ig, iv, ip	Mouse	
81	Myrrha				
82	Natrii sulfas	6.738 g/kg[2]	ip	Mouse	
83	Natrii sulfas exsiccatus				
84	Notoginseng radix et rhizoma	33≥5000 mg/kg[1,2]	ih, ivgtt, ip, po	Mouse	
84	Notoginseng radix et rhizoma	498 mg/kg[1]	ivgtt	Guinea-pig	
85	Olibanum				
86	Persicae semen	222.5 g/kg[2]	ip	Mouse	
87	Physochlainae radix	43 g/kg[2]	ip	Mouse	
88	Polygoni cuspidati rhizoma et radix	249.5–1000 mg/kg[1]	ip	Mouse	
89	Pruni semen				
90	Psammosilenes radix				
91	Rhapontici radix				
92	Rhei radix et rhizoma	0.56–153.5 g/kg[1,2]	po	Mouse	
93	Sappan lignum	18.9 g/kg[2]	ip	Mouse	
94	Selaginellae herba				
95	Sennae folium	1.414 g/kg[1]	ip	Mouse	
96	Sulfur	0.266 g/kg[1]	ig	Mouse	
97	Tetrapanacis medulla				
98	Trichosanthis radix	0.236–2.26 mg/each animal[1]	iH	Mouse	
99	Typhae pollen	35.57 g/kg[2]	ip	Mouse	
100	Typhonii rhizoma	29.57–32.58 g/kg[1,4]	iv	Mouse	
101	Vaccariae semen				
102	Wenyujin rhizoma concisum				

[1]Main component (s).
[2]Herbal water extraction.
[3]Decoction.
[4]Raw herb.
ip: peritoneal injection; ig: intragastrical administration; iv: intravenous injection; iH: hypodermic injection; po: oral administration; im: intramuscular injection.

Table 3. Animal toxicity data of CHMs for pregnancy [15, 16].

5. Conclusions and recommendations

5.1. Chinese medicines are not free of risk

The active ingredients of the Chinese medicines are chemicals that are similar to prescribed drugs. Chinese medicines are not free of risk and they have the same potential to cause adverse effects.

In this overview of Chinese medicines for pregnancy with well-characterized reproductive toxicity, though these Chinese medicines are not commonly used in clinical practice, some of them could result in severe consequences when given in over dosages or even normal dosages. In the communities which use Chinese medicines, special attention should be paid and precautions should be taken to prevent mistaken overdoses of the Chinese medicines.

5.2. International guideline is necessary

It should be acknowledged that some of the studies from animals may not be comparable to human responses, both referring to Chinese medicines and Western medicines. Despite variations in clinical practice and therapeutic prescription, Chinese medication in Traditional Chinese Medicine should comply with modern pharmacological principles as in Western Medicine. Chinese medicines may be beneficial but may also adversely affect both mothers and fetuses in utero. International regulations have not been designed or specified to categorize the Chinese medicines for use in pregnancy. Until now, no detailed/well-designed reproductive toxicity and pharmacotoxicity studies are available to assess the potential risk of Chinese medicines during pregnancy, as much as true that conventional medications are not well tested in pregnancy too.

Before the detailed studies become available, here we take the initiative in gathering information about the adverse effects and potential toxicity of the Chinese medicines for pregnancy from Chinese Pharmacopeia and the extensive literature studies.

5.3. Recommendations

We hope more comprehensive and systematic experiments will be carried out. Until more reliable and scientific research data become available, clinicians should appraise both the risk and benefit before recommendations to pregnant women or women who plan to be pregnant. Both Chinese and Western physicians should explicitly elicit and document the history of the use of any Chinese medications. This is to prevent and recognize potential serious problems associated with their use and should encourage their discontinuation. More studies and clinical trials in humans with a larger sample size are obviously mandatory. We do recommend more systematic basic investigation of the safety use of Chinese medicines for pregnancy.

Acknowledgements

L. L. has received fellowships from Deutscher Akademischer AustauschDienst (DAAD), Research Fellowship Scheme (RFS) and National Natural Science Foundation of China (NSFC) Young Scientist Fund project for her research projects on Chinese herbal medicines in Germany, Hong Kong SAR China and Mainland China, respectively, in 2013 and 2014.

Author details

Lu Li[1, 2], Ling Shan Han[3], Xue Lu Jiang[3], Ping Chung Leung[2, 4] and Chi Chiu Wang[5]*

*Address all correspondence to: ccwang@cuhk.edu.hk

1 College of Basic Medical Sciences, Zhejiang Chinese Medical University, Hangzhou, Zhejiang Province, P. R. China

2 Institute of Chinese Medicine, The Chinese University of Hong Kong, Shatin, New Territories, Hong Kong

3 Department of Obstetrics & Gynaecology, First Affiliated Hospital of Zhejiang Chinese Medical University, Hangzhou, Zhejiang Province, P. R. China

4 State Key Laboratory of Phytochemistry and Plant Resources in West China, The Chinese University of Hong Kong, Shatin, New Territories, Hong Kong

5 Department of Obstetrics & Gynaecology, The Chinese University of Hong Kong, Shatin, New Territories, Hong Kong

References

[1] Li J. In: Formula (Fang Ji Xue). 1st ed. Beijing: China Press of Traditional Chinese Medicine; 2006. pp. 1–30. Ch. 1.

[2] Guo P. In: A Chinese Bestiary—Strange Creatures from the Guideways Through Mountains and Seas (Shan Hai Jing). 1st ed. Changsha: Chang Sha Commercial Press; 1939. pp. 1–15. Ch. 1.

[3] Li JB. In: Chinese Medicine (Zhong Yi Xue). 6th ed. Beijing: People's Health Publishing House; 2005. 300 p.

[4] Ma BZ, Liu RF, Du HL. In: Obstetrics & Gynaecology in Chinese Medicine (Zhong Yi Fu Ke Xue). 6th ed. Shanghai: The Science & Technology Press; 2006. 200 p.

[5] Jiang ZY. Mint: Clinical study of 99 cases of ectopic pregnancy treated with combination of traditional Chinese medicine and Western Medicine. Asia-Pacific Traditional Medicine. 2009;**7**:32–33.

[6] Li CZ. Mint: Observation on the curative effect of conservative treatment of ectopic pregnancy with combined Chinese medicine and Western medicine. Modern Journal of Integrated Chinese Traditional and Western Medicine. 2009;**8**:41–43.

[7] Wang SM, Luo WQ. In: Image of Traditional Chinese Medicine: A Study on the History of Traditional Chinese Medicine. 1st ed. Beijing: People's Medical Publishing House; 2007. 100 p.

[8] Duke JA. Returning to our Medicinal Roots (herbal medicine for alternative health care) [Internet]. 2001. Available from: http://www.highbeam.com/doc/1G1-73088521.html. [Accessed:2016-09-01].

[9] Li L, Leung PC, Wang CC. Efficacy and safety of Chinese medicines for threatened miscarriage. In: Miscarriages: Causes, Symptoms and Prevention. Tranquilli AL Eds. New York, USA: NOVA Publisher;2012. pp. 155–186. Ch. 10.

[10] Li L, Dou LX, Leung PC, Wang CC. Mint: Chinese herbal medicines for threatened miscarriage (Review). Cochrane Database of Systematic Reviews. 2012;5:Art.No.: CD008510. DOI: 10.1002/14651858.CD008510.pub2. pp. 1-86.

[11] Li L, Dou LX, Leung PC, Chung TKH, Wang CC. Chinese herbal medicines for unexplained recurrent miscarriage (Review). Cochrane Database of Systematic Reviews. 2016;1:Art.No.: CD010568. DOI: 10.1002/14651858.CD010568.pub2. pp. 1–44.

[12] Wu K, Chen BQ, Zhang GQ. Mint: Study on toxicity of Gan Sui injection. Ha'er Bin Journal of Harbin Medical University. 1990;**24**(6):484–486.

[13] Li L, Dou LX, James P, Neilson A, Leung PC, Wang CC. Mint: Adverse outcomes of Chinese medicines used for threatened miscarriage: a systematic review and meta-analysis. Human Reproduction Update. 2012;**18**(5):504–524.

[14] Li L, Leung PC, Chung TKH, Wang CC. Chinese herbal medicine for recurrent miscarriage: A systematic review. In: Miscarriages: Diagnosis, Management and Coping Strategies. Pannel VM Eds. New York, USA: NOVA Publisher; 2014. pp. 133–153. Ch. 5.

[15] Zhang W. In: Chinese Pharmacopeia. 10th ed. Beijing: The Medicine Science and Technology Press of China; 2015. 418 p.

[16] Song LR. In: Chinese Materia Medica. 1st ed. Beijing: State Administration of Traditional Chinese Medicine of the People's Republic of China; 1999. 9282 p.

Section 3

Chinese Medical Therapies

Chapter 4

Qigong for the Management of Type 2 Diabetes Mellitus

Guan-Cheng Sun, Catherine Osgood and Harold Ryan Lilly

Additional information is available at the end of the chapter

http://dx.doi.org/10.5772/67065

Abstract

Type 2 diabetes mellitus (T2MD) is a complex, chronic, metabolic disease with hyperglycemia arising from insulin resistance, progressive pancreatic beta cell failure, insufficient insulin secretion and increased hepatic glucose output. In the Chinese medicine theory, T2DM is often referred to as a form of *Xiao Ke* (消渴) or "wasting-thirst disorder." Genetic, dietary, lifestyle and environmental factors play a role in T2DM. People with a family history of diabetes or who are obese are at the highest risk of developing the disease. T2DM is often associated with hypertension, dyslipidemia and atherosclerosis and if not managed can lead to complications including cerebrovascular accident, peripheral vascular disease and nephropathy. T2DM can be well managed with biomedical and Chinese medicine treatment approaches. Lifestyle changes including appropriate diet and exercise are paramount in managing T2DM. Regular Qigong practice can be a beneficial part of one's exercise routine for T2DM self-care. Qigong exercise has shown promising results in clinical experience and in randomized, controlled pilot studies for affecting aspects of T2DM including positive associations between participation in Qigong and blood glucose, triglycerides, total cholesterol, weight, BMI and insulin resistance. This chapter looks at how traditional Chinese medicine (TCM) views diabetes as well as new understandings of how Qigong can support the management of T2DM.

Keywords: medical Qigong, Qigong exercise, type 2 diabetes management, *Xiao Ke*, acupuncture and oriental medicine, traditional Chinese medicine (TCM) nutrition natural medicine, integrative medicine, Yi Ren® Qigong

1. Introduction

Qigong (pronounced "chee gung") is the authentic cultivation of "Qi" (or "Chi") which means "vital energy of the body." In Chinese, "gong" means the skill and achievement cultivated through regular and disciplined practice. Qigong is an important part of traditional Chinese medicine (TCM) for maintaining wellness, preventing disease and treating disease through self-care practice or by receiving external Qi from a Qigong therapist. In ancient China, the practice of authentic Qi cultivation was associated with the theory of energy flow within the body, described in the *Suwen* (Basic Questions) of the *Huangdi Neijing* (The Inner Classic of the Yellow Emperor) and with the discovery of acupuncture meridians as described in the *Ling Shu* (The Spiritual Pivot). The practice of Qigong combines breathing, movement and meditation and therefore is often classified by Western providers under the category of "mind/body medicine." Qigong is an ancient technology of mind-body management and the refinement of one's vital energy for optimal health and for personal development [1]. Previous studies suggest that Qigong may be a beneficial adjunct treatment for individuals with type 2 diabetes mellitus (T2DM) and have shown consistent and statistically significant positive associations between participation in Qigong and blood glucose, triglycerides and total cholesterol [2]. Qigong has also been associated with trends in weight loss, reduced BMI and improved insulin resistance in people with T2DM [3]. Systematic reviews have found support for a role of Qigong in the management of T2DM [4, 5].

T2DM is a complex, chronic metabolic disease with hyperglycemia arising from insulin resistance, progressive pancreatic beta cell failure and insufficient insulin secretion. According to the International Diabetes Federation (IDF), more than 371 million people worldwide have diabetes and over 550 million people are projected to have diabetes by 2030 [6]. In adults, T2DM accounts for about 90–95% of all diagnosed cases of diabetes [7]. Common symptoms of T2DM include excessive thirst, frequent urination, excessive hunger, fatigue, weight loss, blurry vision, slow-healing sores, frequent infections (bacterial, yeast, or fungal overgrowths thrive on excess sugar in the body) and areas of darkened skin, usually in the armpits and neck which can be a sign of insulin resistance [8]. T2DM is often associated with hypertension, dyslipidemia and atherosclerosis and if not managed can lead to complications including stroke, cardiovascular disease, peripheral vascular disease, neuropathy and kidney failure [9]. Concurrent hypertension with diabetes significantly raises the risk of coronary artery disease, stroke, retinopathy and sexual dysfunction [10]. According to the American Diabetes Association, having diabetes nearly doubles the chance of having a heart attack [9]. Diabetes causes more deaths a year in the United States than AIDS and breast cancer combined [11]. In 2010 in the United States alone, about 73,000 lower-limb amputations were performed on adults with diabetes and peripheral vascular disease [12]. T2DM can substantially diminish quality of life, decrease life expectancy and increase health problems and healthcare costs. A study reported that the estimated total economic cost of diagnosed diabetes in 2012 in the United States was $245 billion. This estimate highlights the substantial burden that diabetes imposes on society [13]. The incidence of T2DM continues to rise by epidemic proportions and has emerged as a global health crisis.

2. The pathophysiology and etiology of type 2 diabetes mellitus

The exact cause of T2DM is unknown, but researchers tend to agree that genetic, dietary and lifestyle factors play a role in T2DM [14]. People with a family history of diabetes or who are obese are at the highest risk of developing the disease [8, 9]. Genes associated with T2DM have often been linked to pancreatic beta cells and impairments in beta cell mass and in insulin secretion [15]. The risk of developing T2DM increases when a parent or sibling has the disease [8]. Because population-level genetic changes take many generations to occur, the epidemic proportions of T2DM are almost certainly primarily a consequence of recent environmental changes; nonetheless, T2DM does appear to occur preferentially in genetically predisposed populations, which suggests that the effects of preexisting susceptibility genes have been triggered by recent shifts in nongenetic factors [16]. The environment has great biological impact on human health and disease. There is a growing body of literature suggesting a role for epigenetic factors in the complex interplay between genes and the environment, particularly in common complex disorders, like T2DM [16]. Studies have demonstrated that nutrients can reverse or change epigenetic phenomena such as DNA methylation and histone modifications, thereby modifying the expression of critical genes associated with physiologic and pathologic processes [17].

An improper diet (high in sugar, carbohydrates and fats) and inadequate exercise are contributing factors in the onset of T2DM. The common use of high-fructose corn syrup in foods over the past hundred years has correlated closely with the increasing prevalence of metabolic syndrome, obesity and T2DM, possibly because fructose can alter satiety and lead to the urge to eat more than one ordinarily would [18]. Fructose may also lower metabolism and alter how fat is stored and give rise to the buildup of visceral fat [18]. Fat distribution in the body is important; if fat is stored primarily in the abdomen as opposed to the hips and thighs, there is a higher risk of developing fatty liver, insulin resistance and T2DM [8, 9, 19]. Fatty liver is associated with metabolic syndrome and insulin resistance [9, 19]. One can have fatty liver and not be overweight. If one is overweight and has acquired insulin resistance, losing weight and lowering blood glucose levels through exercise and dietary changes can improve insulin resistance [9, 19]. Exercise is important for regulating one's body weight. Physical activity acts like insulin in that it uses up glucose. Physical activity also makes the body's cells more sensitive to insulin [8].

Obesity is a major risk factor in T2DM because obesity can lead to metabolic disorder and insulin resistance [14]. Many obese people do not develop diabetes, but most people who have T2DM are obese. It is important to point out that people who are not overweight can develop T2DM [11, 15]. Sometimes people who do not appear to have noticeable symptoms may have T2DM and be undiagnosed for many years until complications arise [8]. A high body mass index (BMI) and insulin resistance are primary cofactors in T2DM, but some researchers suggest that the disease could be linked to the pancreatic beta cells themselves, whether due to a reduction in the number of insulin-secreting cells or due to an impairment of beta cell function [15]. In a healthy person, the pancreatic beta cells secrete insulin into the bloodstream and the insulin circulates and enables sugar to enter into the body's cells for the production of energy [8]. Insulin lowers the amount of sugar in the bloodstream and as the sugar level drops, the pancreas also decreases insulin secretion [8]. In T2DM, this process is impaired because as sugar builds up in the bloodstream the pancreatic beta cells release more insulin but over time the beta cells cannot manage the high levels of blood sugar and they start to lose their function [8].

Excess sugar in the blood can affect nerve conductivity by impairing the tiny blood vessels that nourish the nerves leading to neuropathy or sensations of tingling, numbness, burning or pain, especially in the extremities. Over time it can lead to the loss of blood flow to the extremities and develop into gangrene [8]. One of the early signs of nerve and blood vessel damage from T2DM in men is erectile dysfunction [8, 9, 20]. The damage to tiny blood vessels can also lead to retinopathy, blurry vision, eye damage and even blindness [8, 9]. Similarly, high blood glucose levels can injure the delicate blood vessels that make up the filtration system of the kidneys which can lead to irreversible damage and end-stage kidney failure that requires dialysis or a kidney transplant [8, 9].

3. Traditional Chinese medicine (TCM), etiology and pathogenesis of diabetes

In the view of traditional Chinese medicine, the etiology and pathogenesis of diabetes shares much in common with biomedical perspectives. Both traditions recognize that diabetes can arise from one's inherited constitution, which in biomedical terms is linked to one's DNA and in Chinese medicine is understood as one's prenatal or "preheaven essence." In other words, it is the vital energy and "Qi-information" one inherits from one's parents and ancestors as well as the amount of Qi-energy a person is equipped with before birth which carries with it one's potential for health and longevity. The etiology of diabetes can originate with preheaven kidney essence or kidney yin deficiency and weakness of the five zang organs that predispose a person to further imbalances such as spleen Qi deficiency and dampness [20].

Similar to biomedicine, it is important in TCM for practitioners of acupuncture and oriental medicine to think about the digestive function of the pancreas in the treatment of diabetes mellitus [20]. In the TCM theory, what was translated (or perhaps even mistranslated and perpetuated) long ago as "spleen" is often said to more closely resemble the pancreas [3, 21]. TCM explanations of the function of spleen Qi relate to digestion, namely the transportation and transformation of fluids, whereas the biomedical understanding of the spleen has nothing to do with digestion. The biomedical spleen plays a key role in the body's lymphatic and immune system. The TCM concept of spleen Qi actually more appropriately fits "pancreas Qi" and it is the function of the pancreas that is weakened and leads to diabetes [22]. For the purposes of congruency, the term "spleen Qi" can be taken to mean "pancreas Qi" throughout this chapter.

In biomedical and Chinese medicine perspectives, lifestyle behaviors are also important and can trigger diabetes. From a biomedical standpoint, epigenetics plays a role. Behaviors such as overeating of certain foods, environmental factors, a sedentary lifestyle, or the opposite—overtaxing the body with prolonged stress or overexertion, can turn on genes that lead to

T2DM. Chinese medicine perspectives are similar in that "postheaven" choices or lifestyle behaviors can influence the onset and progression of T2DM. Improper diet, overeating of certain foods and overtaxing the body can weaken the Qi-energy and disrupt the balance of the zang (organs). Likewise, a sedentary lifestyle can weaken the Qi because not enough Qi is generated to invest in the strengthening of the body [23].

In Chinese medicine, moderation is key. Too much or too little of any one thing can disrupt Qi flow and balance, so just as a sedentary lifestyle weakens the body because it is too yin, a lifestyle that is too yang with a high level of activity that exceeds the body's resources can also weaken the body [23]. In particular, overworking and not balancing one's energy with enough rest or proper nutrition can deplete the vital energy. Chinese medicine also speaks of overindulgence in sexual activity which weakens the energy of the kidneys and depletes the essence. Prolonged stress and emotional imbalance are also factors that weaken the energy of the organs and the Qi, blood, yin and yang and create disharmony in the body that over time leads to disease.

Chinese medicine often refers to diabetes as Xiao Ke (消 渴), which is translated as "wasting-thirst disorder" and encompasses diabetes mellitus along with other endocrine or metabolic disorders that fit particular patterns with symptoms of a strong appetite and strong thirst (for example, Xiao Ke could refer to other biomedical diseases like hyperthyroidism). Xiao Ke can also refer to stages of diabetes including prediabetes and diabetic complications [20]. In other words, Xiao Ke is a general term which is not the equivalent of diabetes mellitus. Diabetes mellitus is now often referred to using the Chinese modern term Tang Niao Bing (糖尿病) which is literally glucosuria [20].

The diagnosis Xiao Ke Bing, or Xiao Ke Disease, is a group of symptoms related to diabetes that can be further differentiated. The traditional, San Jiao or "three burners" differentiation of Xiao Ke has been popular since the Song Dynasty and is still taught in acupuncture schools as a textbook TCM understanding of diabetes. However, the three burners' differentiation may not be complete, practical, or applicable in clinic now because there are additional symptoms and patterns that should be taken into consideration [20, 24]. Upper (burner) Xiao Ke was traditionally characterized as Xiao Ke with predominant thirst. Middle (burner) Xiao Ke was characterized by excessive appetite and heat and lower (burner) Xiao Ke was characterized by excessive and frequent urination [23]. In modern times, it is important to not give a TCM diagnosis and Xiao Ke differentiation only according to the predominance of excessive thirst, hunger, or urination. It is more appropriate to look closely at the whole body's system, symptoms and patterns and to take into account all the contributing factors including preheaven essence (congenital inheritance), postheaven lifestyle (diet, exercise and stress), as well as one's emotions and environmental stressors.

To provide an overview, the following are some common TCM pattern differentiations associated with T2DM from acupuncture and Chinese herbal medicine treatment perspectives.

The kidney is central to the Chinese medicine understanding of the pathogenesis of T2DM. The kidney stores the jing-essence or one's inherited, original reserves of vital energy. If one has constitutional kidney deficiency, one may already be deficient in yin and may be predisposed to other organ imbalances. This is somewhat similar to saying that one's genes might set them up for epigenetic changes that can be triggered by certain exposures, lifestyle behaviors, or by prolonged stress or emotional imbalances. Overexertion (such as overworking without adequate rest) and overindulgence in sexual activity deplete the kidney yin and jing [25]. A main etiological dynamic in T2DM is kidney yin deficiency at the root which causes dryness heat symptoms as the branch [20, 25]. The relationship between yin deficiency and dryness heat is a circular mechanism because as dryness heat builds, it further consumes the yin fluids [25]. The hyperactive fire resulting from kidney yin deficiency flares upward, resulting in dryness of the lung and heat in the stomach, which combined with kidney yin deficiency, causes diabetes [25].

In addition, chronic kidney yin deficiency can diminish the generation of kidney yang. Combined kidney yin and yang deficiency can in the long run lead to kidney qi failure, making the kidney unable to regulate the exiting of body fluids and manifesting as the need to urinate directly after drinking [26].

In the Chinese medicine theory, the lung is responsible for the descending and distributing of lung Qi and is the upper source of the circulation of water or body fluids [25, 26]. Heat and dryness that consume the yin fluids can injure the lung which then cannot function as well to distribute body fluids and this can present as thirst. Because the lung Qi is responsible for regulating the body's water passages, if lung Qi fails to do this, water and fluid will go directly downward leading to excessive and frequent urination [25, 26].

The liver also plays a central role in the Chinese medicine view of the pathogenesis of T2DM. It is a fairly recent understanding in biomedicine that emotional stress can trigger the onset of T2DM and it is recognized that stress exacerbates high blood glucose levels in people with T2DM [14, 26, 27]. In Chinese medicine theory, the liver is responsible for regulating the smooth flow of Qi throughout the body. Liver Qi stagnation results from stress or excessive emotions and is particularly associated with anger, frustration, irritability, or depression. Constraint and heat from stagnating liver Qi can cause the liver to overact on the middle Jiao which weakens the pancreas Qi and engenders dampness and can also cause too much heat in the stomach, leading to an excessive appetite. Liver Qi stagnation can engender heat in the blood and cause blood stagnation. Blood stagnation impairs fluid distribution and can be accompanied by phlegm stagnation. Heat turns into dryness heat and consumes the yin and can lead to a deficiency of yin in the liver, kidney and stomach [20]. When the yin cannot properly nourish the luo-collaterals, or smaller branches of the body's main meridians, the luo-collaterals can be damaged. In addition, spleen Qi deficiency and the accumulation of dampness or phlegm can lead to the stagnation of phlegm and Blood in the collaterals. Damage of the luo-collaterals manifests as diabetic complications such as hypertension, retinopathy, neuropathy, nephropathy and cardiovascular disease [20].

From a medical Qigong perspective the main causes of T2DM are associated with an imbalanced autonomic nervous system, weakened pancreas energy, low kidney energy and excess energy of the liver. This is based on clinical observation with internal Qi diagnostics, a process in which a trained Qigong practitioner uses medical Qigong techniques to perceive and assess a person's internal Qi-energy flow through the organs and associated meridians.

http://dx.doi.org/10.5772/67065

During a randomized controlled pilot study conducted at Bastyr University in 2010, a particularly striking and common pattern found in patients with T2DM was a disharmony of Qi flow between the liver and pancreas [3]. With medical Qigong subtle energy-based observation, it was very clear to the evaluating medical Qigong practitioner in the 2010 study that the biomedical spleen is not a key player in organ patterns associated with T2DM, but the pancreas and its energy and function are a focal point of the disease. According to five element theory, the phenomenon of the liver (wood element) overpowering or overacting on the pancreas (earth element) [3] was the main dynamic. In addition, an underlying factor observed was a weak kidney or water element. These observations are in alignment with TCM theories about the role of the kidney and yin deficiency affecting the energetic function of other organs. Furthermore, the observation that in many cases of T2DM the role of the liver and its effect on the energetic function of the pancreas emphasizes the impact of stress in modern-day society on the liver energy, whether stress comes from inappropriate diet, lifestyle, the environment, or overwork.

This internal Qi-subtle energy-based observation may provide additional perspectives for TCM therapies for treating T2DM [3]. We have found that Qigong has synergistic effects with other modalities of TCM for treating T2DM. Qigong exercises that focus on boosting kidney and pancreas energy and relieving stress from the liver and autonomic nervous system can be particularly beneficial in managing T2DM [3, 27, 22]. In addition, the self-realization that arises through Qigong self-care practice can help people with T2DM become more aware of the underlying stressors and contributing factors in their condition and to make proactive lifestyle changes.

4. Medical Qigong

Medical Qigong is defined as the system of authentic Qi (vital energy) practice, which empowers the body to heal itself and to facilitate the healing process of others. It involves appropriate management and regulation of all energetic and informational communications and interactions within and without the body in the process of self-healing and healing others. Medical Qigong is another branch of traditional Chinese medicine.

Medical Qigong consists of two aspects of authentic Qi practices, namely internal medical Qigong and external medical Qigong. Internal medical Qigong refers to self-healing and self-care Qigong practice, or Qigong exercises practiced by oneself. Internal medical Qigong exercises include unique breathing methods, movements for specific health conditions, meditations with unique mudras and internal observations with specific energetic codes and images for healing health conditions. External medical Qigong refers to when a medical Qigong practitioner is facilitating the healing process of others. In external Qigong, the medical Qigong practitioner works with his or her client by cleansing and clearing unhealthy Qi, removing blockages or Qi stagnation from the client's energy field to promote healthy internal Qi circulation, or by projecting specific healing Qi into the energy field of the client and directing it to specific areas and systems of the body for restoring internal balance and harmony. The medical Qigong practitioner may also transmit universal healing energy and energetic intelligence to his or her client for improving health conditions and restoring well-being.

4.1. The history and development of medical Qigong

The term "medical Qigong" was made popular by Guizhen Liu in the 1950s and became part of Chinese mainstream culture. Mr. Liu was famous for teaching *nieyang-gong* (innernourishing *qigong*) and at that time medical Qigong became the standard term for healing and improving health conditions with authentic Qi cultivation, regulation and management.

According to historical documents, Qigong has been practiced and studied for about five thousand years in China. The following statement was recorded in the Yellow Emperor's Classic of Internal Medicine, *Suwen* Chapter one: "If your mind is calm and peaceful and able to reach a state of emptiness and you hold your spirit within and your authentic Qi flows easily and freely, how could illness arise?" (The reign of the Yellow emperor was 2690–2590 B.C.). An important part of the Yellow Emperor's Classic of Internal Medicine is the *Ling Shu*–Spiritual Pivot, which contains detailed information about the acupuncture meridians. The acupuncture meridians were discovered by Qigong practitioners in ancient times and can be identified with internal visual and experiential perception.

Lao Zi (601–531 B.C.), the founder or "father" of Daoism mentioned authentic Qi cultivation in his classic *Dao De Jing* (Classic on the Dao of Virtues). He emphasized that the way to obtain health was to "concentrate on authentic Qi cultivation and become more flexible." The famous philosopher Zhuang Zi, in his book *Nan Hua Jing* (third century B.C.), stated that "the immortals' breathing reaches down to their heels and the normal person's breathing to the throat." He emphasized the importance of breathing in the internal cultivation. Up to now, one of the commonly accepted definitions of Qigong is breathing exercise. *Xing Qi* refers to "moving the Qi." An early description of this type of Qigong practice, entitled "The Jade Pendant Inscription on *Xing Qi*" (sixth century B.C.), is shown here in **Figure 1**.

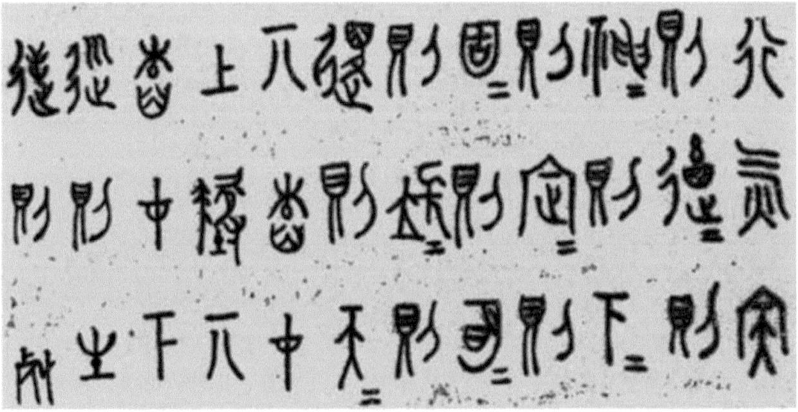

Figure 1. The Jade Pendant Inscription on *Xing Qi* (sixth century B.C.) [28].

The Jade Pendant Inscription on *Xing Qi* could be the earliest monograph on Qigong in Chinese history. It reads as follows:"In moving Qi, one breathes deeply and cultivates the authentic Qi within. If the authentic Qi is stored, it expands. When the authentic Qi expands, it descends down to the Dantian. When the authentic Qi becomes stable in the Dantian, it will solidify. When the authentic Qi is solidified, it will begin to sprout and move to the root of the Du meridian. After the authentic Qi has moved to the root of the Du meridian it will grow and rise up along the Du meridian. When it rises up to the top of the head, it will flow down along the Ren Meridian to the bottom of the torso. When the authentic Qi rises up to the top of the head, it reaches heaven. Heavenly, Qi functions from above and earthly Qi functions from below. Moving the authentic Qi around the Du and Ren meridians freely leads to vitality and longevity while adverseness to this leads to aging and death." *Jing Zuo* literally means"quiet sitting"or"sitting in silence"and refers to a meditation practice to achieve a peaceful and tranquil mind for internal observation, cultivation and realization. Medical Qigong has been practiced with documented results in China. For example, 156 different Qigong therapy methods for healing specific illnesses were described in an ancient book, entitled "Treatise on the Causes and Manifestations of Diseases" (610 A.D.) by Yuan-Fang Chao. In this book, Dr. Chao summarized 1729 cases of diseases from clinical experiences and pathologic observations and explained the symptoms of diseases and their causes as they relate to internal subtle energy flow. For treating diseases, the unique method of Yuan-Fang Chao was to give patients specific Qigong exercises for their self-healing and self-care.

It was during the Jin dynasty (265–420 A.D.) and the northern and southern dynasties (420–589 A.D.) that Qigong developed as a practice to prevent or correct disease through the transmission of healing Qi [29]. A medical Qigong therapist can emit his/her healing Qi to assist another person. This transmitted Qi has healing intelligence that can communicate with another person's Qi for the purpose of addressing specific health conditions [30].

5. The effects of medical Qigong on people with type 2 diabetes

A randomized controlled pilot study was conducted at Bastyr University in 2010 on the effects of Qigong on glucose control in type 2 diabetes [3, 27, 31]. In this study, a three-armed, 12-week randomized, controlled clinical trial compared the biological and psychological responses of Yi Ren Medical Qigong (YRMQ) with progressive resistance training (PRT) or standard care in patients with T2DM. The results on blood glucose control [31], perceived stress [27], body weight and insulin resistance [3] in people with T2DM were interesting and intriguing. Fasting plasma glucose, body weight, body mass index (BMI), insulin and perceived stress levels were recorded before and after the 12-week intervention. As shown in **Figure 2**, the plasma glucose levels indicated significant reductions in the Qigong group. In contrast, the plasma glucose levels showed an increase in both the PRT group and the control group, respectively [31].

The results of the preliminary study showed a very interesting phenomenon as shown in **Figure 3**: the PRT group participants demonstrated significant body weight loss and BMI decrease, but their insulin resistance increased; in contrast, the YRMQ group showed a smaller loss in body weight and BMI, but their insulin resistance decreased [3]. These results suggested that medical Qigong works with a different mechanism for the management of type 2 diabetes compared with PRT [3].

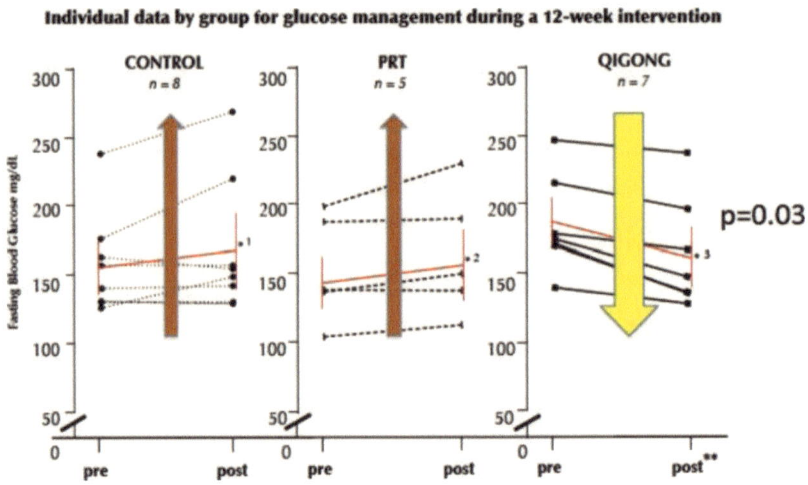

Figure 2. Changes in fasting blood glucose during a 12-week intervention [3, 31].

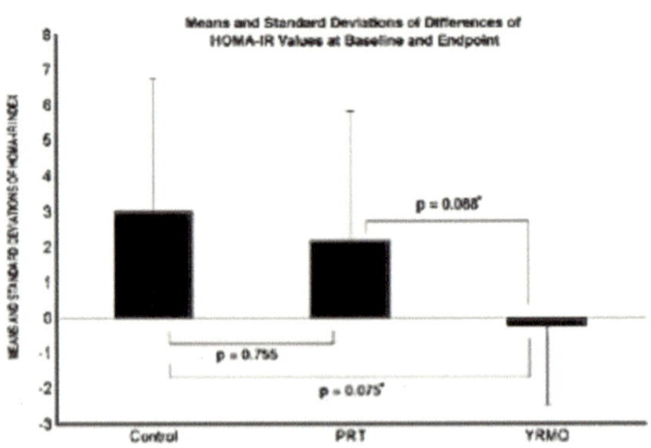

Figure 3. Changes in insulin resistance during a 12-week intervention [3, 31].

Insulin resistance plays a major role in the pathogenesis of metabolic syndrome and T2DM and yet the mechanisms responsible for it remain poorly understood. Current studies have shown that mitochondria may be a major factor in the development of T2DM [32–34]. Mitochondria are known as the powerhouses of the cell. They convert energy from the food that we eat into an energy substance called adenosine triphosphate (ATP) through the process of oxidative respiration. A potential mechanism linking mitochondrial dysfunction to insulin resistance is seen when decreases in substrate oxidation affect electron flow through the electron transport chain (ETC) and lead to the formation of superoxide which damages mitochondria [35]. Mitochondrial superoxide shows evidence of a being a cellular reaction to nutrient excess, leading to insulin resistance with body tissues [36]. Exercise is also known to have a major impact on both mitochondrial function and insulin sensitivity in skeletal muscle [37–40]. Exercise increases energy expenditure and insulin sensitivity. Studies suggest that aerobic exercise may be useful in reversing insulin resistance in prediabetic individuals, possibly preventing the development of type 2 diabetes [34].

One possible explanation for the outcome in the abovementioned study [3] of the YRMQ participants who experienced a reduction in insulin resistance is that in medical Qigong practice, specific Qi-energy breathing exercises that are uniquely recharging might enhance the mitochondrial oxidative respiration process and provide energetic support to mitochondria for preventing ETC electron leakage thereby restoring the functions of the mitochondria for reversing insulin resistance. This possible relationship needs further study.

In addition, it is widely accepted that the etiology of T2DM involves pancreatic β-cell dysfunction and insulin resistance [41]. In molecular genetics studies, the most common mutation leading to mitochondrial diabetes is the A3243G mutation in the mitochondrial encoded tRNA (Leu, UUR) gene [42, 43]. Researchers have found that the A3243G form of mitochondrial diabetes is related to decrease glucose-induced insulin release but is not characterized by insulin resistance, indicating that the major pathology occurs within mitochondria of pancreatic β cells [41]. In the abovementioned study [3], YRMQ group participants practiced, among other Qigong exercises, a specific medical Qigong exercise for empowering the pancreas, which might be beneficial for restoring the functions of the mitochondria of pancreatic β cells. Further studies are needed to investigate these possible benefits.

5.1. Mechanisms of managing type 2 diabetes with medical Qigong

From a medical Qigong perspective, the main cause of T2DM is the imbalance of yin and yang. Another way to look at this is excess sugar intake is too yin and a lack of exercise leads to deficiency of yang. T2DM is largely preventable and many cases could be avoided by lifestyle changes such as eating less and getting appropriate exercise such as walking for 40–60 min/day.

6. Synergistic effects of medical Qigong with acupuncture on type 2 diabetes

Acupuncture and medical Qigong therapy work on the same energetic/Qi "map" of the body, using energy/Qi meridians and points to enhance the body's function in very specific ways. Receiving acupuncture treatments from an experienced Chinese medical practitioner supports the management of T2DM by improving the energetic function of the internal organs.

It must be noted that each individual may present differently and shift presentations over time and the acupuncture and Qigong protocols should be adjusted accordingly for best results. For example, a patient with T2DM and presenting with extreme fatigue, low back and knee pain, excess weight and low motivation may need much more focus on supporting their pancreas and kidneys and less focus on calming down excess energy of the liver. As the patient starts to feel higher energy levels and reduced pain, the acupuncturist might find that the hyperactive liver becomes much more prominent in the patient's presentation and would require an adjustment in the acupuncture treatment and medical Qigong exercises to address the shifting pattern differentiation and to make further progress.

When treating T2DM with acupuncture, practitioners of Chinese medicine may wish to consider two categories of points. The first category consists of points that harmonize and support the zang fu/organ imbalances within the body that are causing the condition. The second group consists of points that help shift unhealthy habits, behaviors and emotions that lead to unhealthy gene expression and diabetes.

From internal Qi-subtle energy-based observation, there are four common areas of zang fu/organ disharmony and dysfunction in the body that must be shifted in order to manage T2DM. These four areas are: (1) excess energy in the liver, (2) low pancreas energy, (3) kidney energy deficiency and (4) an imbalanced autonomic nervous system (represented by the Ren and Du meridians). Although it is important to address all of these imbalances, the key to supporting the successful management of T2DM lies in addressing them at the correct time with each patient:

1. Excess liver (wood element) energy must be released and drained to prevent it from overacting on and damaging the functions of the pancreas (earth element) and affecting the kidneys (water element). Each organ has specific connections with other organs in the body and has the ability to benefit or hinder these relationships. In T2DM, by bringing the liver energy into balance, it sets up the potential for the pancreas and kidneys to recharge and regain normal function. Also, by calming down the liver and creating balance between the liver and the pancreas, the biomedical liver can reduce the amount of glucose it is sending into the bloodstream.

    a. Important points for regulating the Qi and soothing a hyperactive liver: Liver 3, Liver 14, Liver 13, Large Intestine 4 and Large Intestine 10 [23, 44, 45].

2. Low pancreas energy leads to low insulin production and poor blood sugar management. By increasing the energy of the pancreas, its energetic function can improve and play an important part of managing T2DM. By improving the energy of the pancreas, other symptoms can also improve including a reduction in dampness and body weight, reduced fatigue, improved digestive function and less worry and anxiety. This is very important because by improving the pancreas Qi one is working on many different levels including the physiological level (insulin production), the emotional level (decreased worry and anxiety) and the physical level (weight and dampness). In addition, a stronger pancreas will have the energy to keep a potentially hyperactive liver in greater balance.

    a. Important points for increasing the energy of the pancreas: Pancreas 3 (Spleen 3), Pancreas 4 (Spleen 4), Pancreas 6 (Spleen 6), Bladder 20, Bladder 49, Pancreas 9 (Spleen 9), Stomach 36 and Stomach 40 [23, 44, 45].

3. Low kidney energy creates an overall low energetic state in the body and may contribute to insulin resistance. In Chinese medicine, the kidneys are said to be the root of Qi and the foundation of yin and yang in the body [38]. If the foundation of all yin and yang is weak then the rest of the zang fu network can become weak as well. If the root of all the body's energy is increased, the body can return toward its normal function.

   a. Important points for increasing the energy of the kidneys: Kidney 3, Kidney 6, Kidney 7, Bladder 23, Bladder 52 and Pancreas 6 (Spleen 6) [23, 44, 45].

4. An imbalanced autonomic nervous system, from an energetic point of view, is concerned with excess energy expenditure through the sympathetic nervous system without adequate restoration and conservation of energy through the parasympathetic nervous system [46]. In our modern, overstimulated world, many people find it hard to find time to relax and generally operate with an overactivated sympathetic nervous system and constant energy expenditure. This tells the body to send more and more sugar into the bloodstream to bring energy to the cells, causing the pancreas to overwork and the body to become tired. Not only does this affect the body as a whole but it specifically leads to a weakened parasympathetic nervous system that must be restored in order to bring in energy and restore normal functions of the organs.

   a. Important points for balancing the autonomic nervous system: Du 17: stimulates the upper parasympathetic nervous system; Du 2: stimulates the lower parasympathetic nervous system; Lung 7: confluent point of the Ren Meridian; Small Intestine 3: confluent point of the Du Meridian [44].

The second group of points to consider is points that help shift unhealthy habits, emotions and behaviors that contribute to diabetes. These include increased appetite and overeating, emotional and mental health (particularly overthinking, anxiety and worry) and a sedentary lifestyle.

One of the risk factors in T2DM is overeating. An important contribution of acupuncture is to reduce appetite and prevent overeating. Points to reduce appetite and overeating include: Stomach 44, Ren 12, appetite/hunger-control point on the ear.

Points to transform and decrease dampness are very important because dampness by nature makes one feel heavy, tired and stagnant [47]. By transforming dampness, one can feel lighter with increased energy and the desire to be less sedentary. Points include: Pancreas 9 and Stomach 40.

Points for reducing anxiety, worry and overthinking: Du 17, Heart 7 and Ren 17.

7. Western and Chinese medicine nutrition and food restrictions for diabetes

Maintaining healthy target blood glucose levels is key in managing T2DM. Integrative health care, along with self-care through wise food choices, appropriate physical exercise and medical Qigong is a synergistic approach to managing T2DM that can lead to better quality of health and better quality of life.

It is important to work with one's primary care physician to monitor one's A1c and to determine one's target blood glucose levels [48]. Working with a nutritionist to select an appropriate diet and with a Chinese medicine practitioner for support with specific Chinese medicine nutritional recommendations, acupuncture and Chinese herbal medicine that fits one's pattern differentiation, is a holistic approach that can bring more balance to the body. Qi cultivation through the practice of medical Qigong self-care exercises can increase one's vitality and internal, energetic awareness to help a person make dietary and lifestyle changes toward better health.

Generally in both western nutrition and in Chinese medicine nutrition, recommendations for healthy eating for people with T2DM include eating a variety of healthy foods in regular meals while being mindful of portion sizes [49]. Eating small meals at regular times helps to regulate blood sugar and to avoid high spikes in glucose levels after a big meal followed by a drop in blood sugar if a meal is skipped.

The U.S. Department of Health and Human Services and the National Institute of Diabetes and Digestive and Kidney Diseases (NIDDK) offer helpful guidelines entitled "Diabetes Diet and Eating" with suggestions about what to eat, how much to eat and when to eat and they also recommend to those with T2DM to take any necessary medications prescribed by their primary care physicians in order to keep diabetes in check and to prevent diabetic complications [48].

An approach currently being studied by researchers is the very low-calorie diet (VLCD) and its potential to reverse T2DM [50]. A prospective, longitudinal, single-center study published in 2016 showed that people with T2DM who followed a VLCD with total energy intake at 624–700 kcal/day for 8 weeks achieved fasting blood glucose of <7 mmol/L and continuing remission of diabetes for at least 6 months [50]. Data suggests a potential for the reversal of T2DM; however, questions remain about the possibility of long-term, sustained recovery from diabetes [19, 50].

From a Chinese medicine perspective, in addition to moderating portion sizes in order to not overeat, moderation in diet also involves the careful harmonization of the five tastes (sweet, salty, sour, bitter and pungent) and the selection of as much balanced variety as possible in one's daily diet [23]. The more colors one sees on one's plate, the more likely it is that the meal is meeting the nutritional needs of all the organs. It is generally advisable to avoid eating the same foods over and over again because one can miss out on important nutritional benefits that come with eating a diverse range of foods. In addition, the overeating of certain foods leads to imbalances. Eating too many sweet foods damages the spleen (pancreas). Overeating salty foods damages the kidneys and the heart. Eating too many pungent or acrid and spicy foods leads to internal heat which consumes the yin and can worsen diabetes [23].

Food prohibitions in Chinese medicine are focused on not exacerbating a person's specific pattern differentiation [23]. For example, someone with spleen (pancreas) Qi deficiency and dampness would be encouraged to limit or avoid sugar, fatty foods, dairy, raw foods, cold foods and cold drinks in general (e.g., cold salads, smoothies) and instead to have cooked foods like whole grains such as Job's tears, barley, brown rice, millet, quinoa and teff, proteins that are lean, cooked vegetables rather than cold salads and to drink warm liquids in order to aid digestion.

If a person has too much heat in the stomach, foods that are hot in nature should be avoided such as chillies, lamb, alcohol, coffee, garlic and onions [25]. When there is yin deficiency, one should also take care to not eat foods that are overly hot or overly cold or overly drying [25]. If a person has Qi and blood stagnation, foods that are overly cloying, heavy, or difficult to digest should be avoided because they can worsen stagnation. Overeating and emotional eating can also cause stagnation, so a relaxed and positive frame of mind is important while eating [47]. One should avoid eating when feeling irritable or angry, eating while working or multitasking, eating on the run, or eating heavy meals late in the day, or eating too late at night in order to prevent stagnation [47]. It is helpful to eat the main meal earlier in the day to allow adequate time for optimal digestion and to make mealtime a peaceful time for the benefit of all the organs [47]. In the evening, the body's organs naturally start to transition into a rest and restore mode and eating late at night disrupts this process and weakens organ function. If one is hungry late at night, a light, low-carbohydrate, sugar-free and protein-rich snack such as a handful of seeds and a warm glass of water or hot herbal tea can curb hunger and prevent a glucose spike [20].

7.1. TCM food for diabetes management

Chinese medicine food therapy for managing T2DM includes a very special food that doubles as a Chinese herb: *Ku Gua*, known as bitter melon or bitter gourd (Fructus Momordicae Charantiae). It has been used since ancient times in China, India and other parts of the world in the management of what we now call diabetes. Bitter melon contains antidiabetic substances: charantin which reduces blood glucose levels and polypeptide-p which is an insulin-like compound [51]. In Chinese medicine nutrition theory, bitter melon is considered to be bitter and cold and enters the spleen (pancreas), stomach and heart channels. Since bitter melon is thermally cold, people with pancreas Qi deficiency should be mindful to not overeat it since overeating cold foods can further diminish pancreas Qi. However, by adding warming ingredients (e.g., curry seasoning, chili powder and mustard seeds), savory dishes can be prepared that are less cold for the pancreas. For people with excess stomach heat, bitter melon clears stomach heat and by doing so also reduces excessive appetite and can aid in weight loss. Bitter melon can be consumed daily (250–300 g/day) as a juice or by boiling slices of it for several minutes and drinking the water as a tea [20]. People who are taking insulin should use caution when consuming bitter melon because of its additional effect on lowering blood glucose levels.

8. Conclusion

Qigong exercise has shown promising results in clinical experience and in randomized, controlled pilot studies for affecting aspects of T2DM including positive associations between participation in Qigong and blood glucose, triglycerides, total cholesterol, weight, BMI and insulin resistance. Lifestyle changes with appropriate diet and exercise are paramount in managing T2DM. Regular Qigong practice as part of one's exercise routine can have a positive influence on one's awareness of behaviors that either contribute to or improve one's condition and can lead to helpful lifestyle changes, an overall sense of well-being and better health. Qigong exercises can play an important, synergistic role in integrative care with biomedical approaches and with acupuncture, Chinese herbal medicine and nutrition for managing T2DM.

Author details

Guan-Cheng Sun[1], Catherine Osgood[2]* and Harold Ryan Lilly[1]

*Address all correspondence to: gsun@iqim.org

1 Institute of Qigong & Integrative Medicine, Bothell, WA, USA

2 Oregon College of Oriental Medicine, DAOM Program, Class of 2017, Portland, OR, USA

References

[1] Liu T, Chen KW. Chinese Medical Qigong. Singing Dragon. 2010 (ISBN 978 1 84819 023 8):209.

[2] Xin Liu, Yvette D. Miller, Wendy J. Brown. A qualitative review of the role of qigong in the management of diabetes. Journal of Alternative and Complementary Medicine. 2007;13(4):427–33. Epub 2007/05/30.

[3] Guan-Cheng Sun, Xiaobo Ding, Xiao-Hua Zhou, Amy Putiri and Ryan Bradley. Effects of Yi Ren Medical Qigong on body weight in people with Type 2 diabetes mellitus: a secondary analysis of a randomized controlled pilot study. Journal of Integrative Medicine & Therapy. 2014;1(1):1–5.

[4] Lee MS, Chen KW, Choi TY, Ernst E. Qigong for type 2 diabetes care: a systematic review. Complementary Therapies in Medicine. 2009;17(4):236–42. Epub 2009/07/28.

[5] Chen KW, Liu T, Zhang H, Lin Z. An analytical review of the Chinese literature on Qigong therapy for diabetes mellitus. The American Journal of Chinese Medicine. 2009;37(3):439–57. Epub 2009/07/17.

[6] IDF. Type 2 diabetes statistics. http://wwwdiabetescouk/type2-diabeteshtml; 2016.

[7] Ogbera AO, Ekpebegh C. Diabetes mellitus in Nigeria: the past, present and future. World Journal of Diabetes. 2014;5(6):905–11. Epub 2014/12/17.

[8] Staff MC. Type 2 diabetes: symptoms & causes [Internet]. http://wwwmayoclinicorg/diseases-conditions/type-2-diabetes/symptoms-causes/dxc-20169861; 2016.

[9] Maxine Papadakis, Stephen McPhee. Current medical diagnosis & treatment. In: Current Medical Diagnosis & Treatment, 54th edition. New York: McGraw-Hill Education. 2015.

[10] Lago RM, Singh PP, Nesto RW. Diabetes and hypertension. Nature Clinical Practice Endocrinology & Metabolism. 2007;3(10):667. Epub 2007/09/26.

[11] Association AD. Diabetes Myths. http://wwwdiabetesorg/diabetes-basics/myths/; 2016.

[12] Association AD. Statistics about Diabetes. http://wwwdiabetesorg/diabetes-basics/statistics/ 2016;cited 2016 Jul 21.

[13] American Diabetes Association. Economic costs of diabetes in the U.S. in 2012. Diabetes Care. 2013;36(4):1033–46. Epub 2013/03/08.

[14] Blair M. Diabetes mellitus review. Urologic Nursing. 2016;36(1):27–36. Epub 2016/04/21.

[15] Meier JJ, Bonadonna RC. Role of reduced beta-cell mass versus impaired beta-cell function in the pathogenesis of type 2 diabetes. Diabetes Care. 2013;36(Suppl 2):S113–S9. Epub 2013/08/02.

[16] Ling C, Groop L. Epigenetics: a molecular link between environmental factors and type 2 diabetes. Diabetes. 2009;58(12):2718–25. Epub 2009/11/27.

[17] Choi SW, Friso S. Epigenetics: a new bridge between nutrition and health. Advances in Nutrition. 2010;1(1):8–16. Epub 2011/11/02.

[18] Johnson RJ, Nakagawa T, Sanchez-Lozada LG, Shafiu M, Sundaram S, Le M, et al. Sugar, uric acid and the etiology of diabetes and obesity. Diabetes. 2013;62(10):3307–15. Epub 2013/09/26.

[19] Taylor R. Type 2 diabetes: etiology and reversibility. Diabetes Care. 2013;36(4):1047–55. Epub 2013/03/23.

[20] Lu Z. Dr. Zhaoxue Lu's Presentation on Diabetes at OCOM. PowerPoint Presentation for Doctoral Students Oregon College of Oriental Medicine. 2016;May 7.

[21] Dan Bensky. Purpose 志, Elation 喜 and the Pancreas 脾. Medical Acupuncture https://wwwjadeinstitutecom/jade/purpose-elation-pancreasphp 1992;cited 2016 Aug 11.

[22] Sun G-C. Cultivating the body's information system and experiencing the meridians through Qigong practice. Qi, The Journal of Traditional Eastern Health and Fitness. 2004;14(1):22–9.

[23] Bob Flaws, Lynn Kuchinski, Robert Casanas. The Treatment of Diabetes Mellitus with Chinese Medicine. A Textbook and Clinical Manual, 1st edition. Boulder, CO: Blue Poppy Press. 2002.

[24] An Ying Jun. Experience on differentiation and treatment of diabetes. New England Journal of Traditional Chinese Medicine. 2004;Summer(1(3)):25–7.

[25] Ouyang Bing, Gu Zhen. Traditional Chinese Medicine Treatment and Dietetic Restraint for Common Diseases, 1st edition. Jinan, China: Shandong Science and Technology Press. 1995.

[26] William Chi-Shing Cho, Kevin Kin-Man Yue, Albert Wing-Nang Lueng. An outline of diabetes mellitus and its treatment by traditional Chinese medicine and acupuncture. The Journal of Chinese Medicine. Jun 2005;(78):33–41.

[27] Putiri AL, Lovejoy JC, Gillham S, Sasagawa M, Bradley R, Sun GC. Psychological effects of Yi Ren Medical Qigong and progressive resistance training in adults with type 2 diabetes mellitus: a randomized controlled pilot study. Alternative Therapies in Health and Medicine. 2012;18(1):30–4. Epub 2012/04/21.

[28] Association CMQ. What is Inscription on Xing Qi (in Chinese). http://wwwcmqgcn/science/science009html 2016.

[29] Xu X. History of Qigong. http://wwwinnerselfcom/Fitness/qigong_historyhtm. 2012.

[30] Kenneth M. Sancier and Linda Hole. Qigong and neurologic illness. Qigong Institute. http://www.qigonginstitute.org/docs/Qig ong&Neurologic_Illness.pdf

[31] Sun GC, Lovejoy JC, Gillham S, Putiri A, Sasagawa M, Bradley R. Effects of Qigong on glucose control in type 2 diabetes: a randomized controlled pilot study. Diabetes Care. 2010;33(1):e8. Epub 2009/12/31.

[32] Yi Lin and Zhongjie Sun. Current views on type 2 diabetes. The Journal of Endocrinology. 2010;204(1):doi:10.1677/JOE-09-0260.

[33] Mary-Elizabeth Patti and Silvia Corvera. The role of mitochondria in the pathogenesis of type 2 diabetes. Endocrine Reviews. 2010;31(3):364–95.

[34] Rebecca Parish and Kitt Falk Petersen. Mitochondrial dysfunction and type 2 diabetes. Current Diabetes Reports. 2005;5(3):177–83.

[35] Magdalene K Montgomery and Nigel Turner. Mitochondrial dysfunction and insulin resistance: an update. Endocrine Connections. 2015;4:R1–R15.

[36] Kyle L. Hoehn, Adam B. Salmon, Cordula Hohnen-Behrens, Nigel Turner, Andrew J. Hoy, Ghassan J. Maghzal, Roland Stocker, Holly Van Remmen, Edward W. Kraegen, Greg J. Cooney, Arlan R. Richardson, and David E. James. Insulin resistance is a cellular antioxidant defense mechanism. Proceedings of the National Academy of Sciences of the United States of America. 2009;106(42):17787–92.

[37] Phielix E MR, Moonen-Kornips E, Hesselink MK, Schrauwen P. Exercise training increases mitochondrial content and ex vivo mitochondrial function similarly in patients with type 2 diabetes and in control individuals. Diabetologia. 2010;53:1714–21.

[38] Toledo FG ME, Ritov VB, Azuma K, Radikova Z, DeLany J, DE. K. Effects of physical activity and weight loss on skeletal muscle mitochondria and relationship with glucose control in type 2 diabetes. Diabetes. 2007;56:2142–7.

[39] Joachim Nielsen, Martin Mogensen, Birgitte F. Vind, Kent Sahlin, Kurt Højlund, Henrik D. Schrøder, Niels Ørtenblad. Increased subsarcolemmal lipids in type 2 diabetes: effect of training on localization of lipids, mitochondria and glycogen in sedentary human skeletal muscle. American Journal of Physiology, Endocrinology and Metabolism. 2010;298:E706–E71.

[40] Ruth C.R. Meex, Vera B. Schrauwen-Hinderling, Esther Moonen-Kornips, Gert Schaart, Marco Mensink, Esther Phielix, Tineke van de Weijer, Jean-Pierre Sels, Patrick Schrauwen, and Matthijs K.C. Hesselink. Restoration of muscle mitochondrial function and metabolic flexibility in type 2 diabetes by exercise training is paralleled by increased myocellular fat storage and improved insulin sensitivity. Diabetes. 2010;59:572–9.

[41] William I. Sivitz and Mark A. Yorek. Mitochondrial dysfunction in diabetes: from molecular mechanisms to functional significance and therapeutic opportunities. Antioxidants & Redox Signaling. 2010;12(4):537–577.

[42] Maassen JA LT, Van Essen E, Heine RJ, Nijpels G, Jahangir Tafrechi RS, Raap AK, Janssen GM, Lemkes HH. Mitochondrial diabetes: molecular mechanisms and clinical presentation. Diabetes. 2004;53(1):S103–S9.

[43] Maassen JA HL, Janssen GM, Reiling E, Romijn JA, Lemkes HH. Mitochondrial diabetes and its lessons for common type 2 diabetes. Biochemical Society Transactions. 2006;34:819–23.

[44] Kim H VLC, Darnell R. Minibook of Oriental Medicine, Charleston, WV: Acupuncture-Mediacom. 2009.

[45] Subhuti Dharmananda. Treatment of Diabetes with Chinese Herbs and Acupuncture: Lowering Blood Sugar http://wwwitmonlineorg/journal/arts/diabeteshtm 2016;cited 22 August 2016.

[46] Guan-Cheng Sun, Jill Gonet. Yi Ren Medical Qigong Manual Volume 1. Seattle: Yi Ren Press. 2013.

[47] Daverick Leggett. Helping Ourselves: A Guide to Traditional Chinese Food Energetics. Totnes, England: Meridian Press. 2014.

[48] National Institute of Diabetes and Digestive and Kidney Diseases (NIDDK). What I need to know about Eating and Diabetes. https://wwwniddknihgov/health-information/diabetes/diabetes-diet-eating. 2016;cited 2016 Aug 11.

[49] American Diabetes Association. Diabetes Meal Plans and a Healthy Diet: What is a Diabetes Meal Plan? . http://wwwdiabetesorg/food-and-fitness/food/planning-meals/diabetes-meal-plans-and-a-healthy-diethtml?loc=ff-slabnav. 2016;cited 2016 Aug 11.

[50] Steven S, Hollingsworth KG, Al-Mrabeh A, Avery L, Aribisala B, Caslake M, et al. Very low-calorie diet and 6 months of weight stability in Type 2 diabetes: pathophysiological changes in responders and nonresponders. Diabetes Care. 2016;39(5):808–15. Epub 2016/03/24.

[51] Diabetes.co.uk the global diabetes community. Bitter Melon and Diabetes. http://wwwdiabetescouk/natural-therapies/bitter-melonhtml. 2016;cited 2016 Aug 16.

Chapter 5

Complementary and Alternative Therapy with Traditional Chinese Medicine for Infertility

Yen-Nung Liao, Wen-Long Hu and Yu-Chiang Hung

Additional information is available at the end of the chapter

http://dx.doi.org/10.5772/66971

Abstract

Infertility results in a country with a low birth rate and an aging population, and thus there is vested interest in treating this problem by using both complementary and alternative therapies, in addition to conventional western medicine. Traditional Chinese medicine (TCM) has been widely used for healthcare in the Eastern world for thousands of years. This chapter describes the evidence to support the role of TCM in the management of male and female infertility.

Keywords: complementary and alternative therapy, traditional Chinese medicine, acupuncture and moxibustion, infertility

1. Introduction

1.1. Definition

Normal fertility was previously defined as the ability to conceive within 2 years of regular unprotected sexual intercourse [1, 2]. Recently, infertility has been defined as failure to conceive within 1 year of regular unprotected sexual intercourse in women less than 35 years old, or within 6 months of unprotected sexual intercourse in women older than 35 years old [2, 3].

1.2. Epidemiology

According to a World Health Organization (WHO) report, the prevalence of infertility has increased since 1990, and the most recent data from 2010 estimated the worldwide incidence of infertile couples to be approximately 48.5 million (**Figure 1**) [4]. In the United States, the percentage of married women aged 15–44 years old who were infertile decreased from 8.5% in 1982 (2.4 million women) to 6.0% (1.5 million) in 2006–2010 [5]. In Taiwan, the total female fertility rate decreased from 7.04 million in 1951 to 1.175 million in 2015 [6]. Taiwan has thus become one of the countries with the lowest fertility rates in the world. In China, the 1- and 2-year infertility rates in newly married couples were 12.5 and 6.6%, respectively [7]. In 2004, a WHO evaluation of Demographic and Health Surveys (DHS) data estimated that more than 186 million ever-married women of reproductive age were infertile, translating into one in every four couples [8].

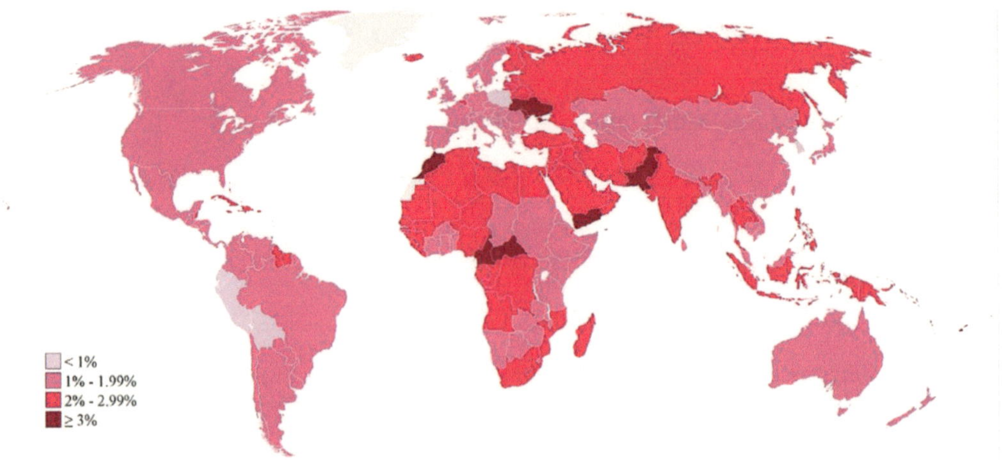

Figure 1. Worldwide prevalence of primary female infertility (2010). Infertility prevalence is indexed based on the age of the female partner; age-standardized prevalence among women aged 20–44 years old is shown here [4].

1.3. Impact

A low fertility rate results in a low birth rate and an aging country. According to the Taiwan Population Policy White Paper, the total population of Taiwan is expected to decrease after 2022 [9]. A review showed that infertility or subfertility is associated with intimate partner violence (IPV) in low- and middle-income countries (LMICs) [10]. Certain fertility treatments may increase the risk of ovarian or breast cancer [11, 12], while others have poor pharmacological efficacy in infertile women older than 40 years [13]. Around one-fifth of all subfertile couples seeking fertility treatment have clinically significant levels of depression, anxiety, and suffering, but the effects of educational and psychological interventions on mental health outcomes and pregnancy outcomes including distress, and live birth or ongoing pregnancy rates, is unclear owing to the very low quality of evidence [14].

2. Etiology

Around 15% of couples have difficulty conceiving [15]. The etiology of infertility can be broadly classified into female- and male-related factors. Among distinguishable female factors, which are responsible for 81% of female infertility, the most common are ovulatory disorders (25%), endometriosis (15%), pelvic adhesions (12%), tubal blockage (11%), other tubal abnormalities (11%), and hyperprolactinemia (7%) [16]. Male factor infertility affects around 30–55% of all couples and is the most difficult form of infertility to treat [17]. The causes of male infertility include environmental disruptors, genetic defects, physiological and endocrine failure, and testicular pathologies [18].

According to the theory of traditional Chinese medicine, syndromes of female infertility can be classified as the following: kidney deficiency, stagnation of liver qi, static blood blocking in uterine, and accumulation of phlegm-wetness in the body. Constitution has a great effect on the syndrome patterns of many diseases including infertility. A report showed that the constitution ratio of yang deficiency, phlegm damp, and yin deficiency was 29.5, 20.0, and 21.0%, respectively, in sterility patients [19]. This report also pointed that kidney deficiency syndrome was positively correlated with yin deficiency and yang deficiency constitution, blood stasis syndrome was positively associated with blood stasis and yang deficiency constitution, and liver stagnation syndrome was positively correlated with phlegm damp and damp heat constitution.

2.1. Ovulatory disorders

A history of regular menses with molimina (breast tenderness, bloating, cramping, mood changes) is suggestive of ovulation in the majority (95%) of women [20]. Anovulation and oligo-ovulation lead to infertility because an oocyte is not available every month for fertilization. A woman's fecundability reaches a peak in her late-twenties and decreases with advancing age, with a more rapid decline after her mid-thirties [21]. Ovarian ageing causes a progressive loss of the finite pool of primordial follicles and a decrease in the quality of oocytes, mainly because of the accumulation of chromosomal abnormalities [22]. Polycystic ovarian syndrome (PCOS) is a common ovulatory disorder, and patients with this diagnosis are often obese and oligomenorrheic. They tend to have difficulty conceiving owing to ovulatory dysfunction as well as poor oocyte quality and endometrial receptivity [23]. However, the results of epidemiologic data obtained mainly from comparative studies and cohorts, have concluded that the role and size (<6 cm) of ovary cysts in infertility is controversial [24].

2.2. Endometriosis

The rate of infertility among women with endometriosis ranges from 30 to 50%, and dysfunction is due to various mechanisms including pelvic adhesions, abnormal tubal transport, implantation defects, and intraperitoneal inflammation, which can decrease oocyte quality or oocyte-sperm interactions [25].

2.3. Pelvic adhesions

Most adhesions occur after surgical procedures, but can also occur following infection, ischemia, endometriosis, or reaction to a foreign body, and these cause infertility by distorting pelvic anatomy and by blocking the fallopian tubes [26]. Peritubal adhesions negatively affect ovum transportation, while periovarian adhesions inhibit ovum release and ovulatory function [27, 28].

2.4. Tubal blockage and other tubal abnormalities

Tubal anomalies that contribute to infertility include congenital absence and major diverticula, duplication of the tubes, tubal occlusion, and hydrosalpinx [29, 30]. Other causes of tubal infertility include endometriosis, intrauterine contraceptive devices, infections (gonorrhea, chlamydia trachomatis, and genital tuberculosis), and postoperative complications of abdominal surgery [31].

2.5. Hyperprolactinemia

Symptoms of hyperprolactinemia include amenorrhea, oligomenorrhea, infertility, decreased sexual desire, and habitual abortion. Women may also have signs of chronic hyperandrogenism such as acne and hirsutism, which may be related to increasing dehydroepiandrosterone sulfate (DHEAS) secretion from the adrenal glands [32].

3. Diagnosis

History taking and physical examination are paramount to understanding the etiology of the infertility, and should be undertaken in both partners after 1 year of trying to conceive. In certain cases, investigation is indicated after 6 months of unprotected intercourse, such as when the female partner is over 35 years old or has a history of oligomenorrhea or amenorrhea, known or suspected endometriosis or tubal disorders, a past history of chemotherapy or radiation therapy, and in couples in which the male partner is known to be subfertile.

3.1. History taking

A menstrual history (menstrual interval and characteristics) should be elicited in all female patients in order to understand their ovulatory cycles. For instance, regular monthly cycles with premenstrual symptoms (breast tenderness, ovulatory pain, bloating) suggest that the patient is ovulating, whereas severe dysmenorrhea may indicate endometriosis.

A personal and lifestyle history should also be obtained from all infertile couples, including details about occupations; ages; stressors; levels of exercise; diets; and consumption of alcohol, tobacco, and other substances which can influence fertility [33]. It is also important to take a sexual history, including an evaluation of the frequency of intercourse and of underlying problems such as sexual dysfunction. Infrequent or inappropriately timed sexual intercourse can result in infertility.

Clinicians should elicit a full medical, surgical, and obstetric history including information about the number of previous pregnancies, type and number of deliveries, and number of abortions (including spontaneous and induced) [32]. A gynecological history should evaluate any history of pelvic inflammatory disease, sexually transmitted infections, and treatment of abnormal pap smears, as well as uncover any history of procedures or medications, which could be related to infertility. In addition, a review of systems should be conducted in order to evaluate whether a patient has symptoms of dyspareunia, hypo-/hyperthyroidism, pelvic or abdominal pain, galactorrhea, or hirsutism [34].

http://dx.doi.org/10.5772/66971

A family history of infertile couples should record in detail whether any family members have birth defects, mental retardation, genetic mutations, or fertility issues. The most common inherited cause of infertility is fragile X syndrome, which presents as premature ovarian failure (POF) in women, and which can lead to developmental delay or learning problems in men [35].

3.2. Physical examination

The physical examination can uncover signs indicative of latent causes of infertility. The patient's body mass index (BMI) and fat distribution should be measured and calculated, as an abnormally low BMI is related to infertility, whereas abdominal obesity is associated with insulin resistance [34].

In women, the presence of vaginal and cervical discharge or anatomic abnormalities may indicate an underlying infection or Müllerian anomaly, respectively. If the uterus is enlarged, irregular, or lacks mobility, this may suggest the presence of a uterine abnormality such as endometriosis, leiomyoma, or pelvic adhesions. Chronic pelvic inflammatory disease or endometriosis presents with tenderness, or with masses in the adnexa or posterior cul-de-sac (pouch of Douglas), while endometriosis also has palpable tender nodules at the rectovaginal septum or uterosacral ligaments [35].

Patients with Turner syndrome have absent periods, and distinctive morphological features including a squarely shaped chest, and a stocky, short body habitus. Those with hypogonadotropic hypogonadism have primary amenorrhea and unremarkable secondary sexual characteristics. The presence of galactorrhea, thyroid gland anomalies, or signs of androgen excess such as acne, hirsutism, virilization, and male pattern baldness indicate an endocrinopathy (e.g., polycystic ovarian syndrome, adrenal disorders, hyper- or hypothyroidism, hyperprolactinemia) [33, 35].

In men, anatomic abnormalities or discharge from the penis, scrotum, and urethral meatus may indicate the presence of an inguinal/femoral/scrotal hernia, cryptorchidism, or infection. Varicoceles, usually noted on the left side, are associated with infertility, whereas small, hard testes (<2 cm long) are suggestive of Klinefelter's syndrome [36].

3.3. Other diagnostic methods

Additional essential infertility evaluations include semen analyses, assessment of ovulatory function by laboratory tests, and a hysterosalpingogram to uncover underlying uterine abnormalities and evaluate tubal patency.

Diagnostic laparoscopy is recommended for women with suspected pelvic adhesions or endometriosis, during which chromotubation can assess tubal patency and hysteroscopy can assess the uterine cavity [29, 30].

Women older than 35 years and those younger but with risk factors for POF should measure estradiol and follicle-stimulating hormone (FSH) levels on day 3 in order to evaluate the ovarian reserve. Other tests such as antral follicle count, level of anti-Müllerian hormone (AMH), and the clomiphene citrate challenge test (CCCT) should be performed if necessary [35].

4. Conventional treatments and limitations

Assisted reproductive technology (ART), such as artificial insemination (AI), *in vitro* fertilization and embryo transfer (IVF-ET), and intracytoplasmic sperm injection (ICSI), is responsible for up to 4% of infants born in developing countries.

ART has several iatrogenic complications including the risk of multiples, low luteal phase insufficiency, disabled embryo implantation, ovarian hyperstimulation syndrome (OHSS), and other perinatal and long-term health conditions [37]. Furthermore, fertility treatments, especially IVF-ET and ICSI, are costly and risky [38].

Intra-uterine insemination (IUI), one form of AI, is a commonly used fertility treatment for couples with cervical factor infertility, unexplained subfertility, and subfertility in women with endometriosis after surgical resection [39]. IUI is more useful in some types of severe sexual dysfunction such a severe ejaculatory dysfunction or vaginismus; in cases of cervical factor or mild male factor infertility; and to prevent the transmission of sexually transmitted diseases such as hepatitis B/C virus (HBV/HCV) and human immunodeficiency virus (HIV) [40].

It is a relatively simple surgical procedure whereby semen that has been washed in the laboratory is inserted into the uterine cavity by using a small catheter at the time of ovulation. IUI allows sperm to bypass the potentially hostile cervix, and thus increases the number of sperm that reach the uterine cavity and oocyte [40]. The technique can be performed either with or without added medications to encourage ovarian hyperstimulation (OH). In the latter method, follicular growth is monitored either via regular ultrasound monitoring to visualize the follicles or by measuring the preovulatory luteinizing hormone level rise in the serum or urine. In the former, ovulation is induced by an injection of human chorionic gonadotropin (hCG). Timed intercourse (TI), a less invasive method than IUI, involves giving couples information about cycle monitoring so that they can time intercourse appropriately.

Nevertheless, a systematic review revealed that there is no difference in live birth or multiple pregnancy rates in most couples with unexplained subfertility treated with either IUI or TI, both with and without OH [39].

5. Traditional Chinese medicine

Traditional Chinese medicine (TCM) formulas have been used to treat female and male infertility for hundreds of years. Classically, the TCM formulas are combined with several single herbs to treat a specific disease. Some of the single herbs that have been used in women include Semen Cuscutae, Semen Lantaginis, Herba Leonuri Japonici, and Fructus Ligustri Lucidi, and were first recorded in the Chinese classic Shi Jing (the Book of Songs) over 2000 years ago.

5.1. Female infertility

The results of one systematic review revealed that treatment with Chinese herbal medicine can increase pregnancy rates 2-fold in a 4-month period compared to western fertility drugs or IVF [41]. This report also stated that evaluating the quality of the menstrual cycle is essential in order to effectively treat female infertility by TCM. However, in a recent well-controlled clinical trial, there was no significant difference in fertility outcomes after laparoscopy between women with minimal/mild endometriosis treated with oral contraceptives (OC), or OC and Dan&e mixture (composed of six herbs) [42]. A study from the National Health Insurance Research Database (NHIRD) in Taiwan has revealed the most commonly used TCM formulas for the management of female infertility [43]. At the top of the list are Dang-Gui-Sha-Yao-San and Wen-Jing-Tang; the former is used for abdominal pain during pregnancy, while the latter is used for dysmenorrhea and infertility, and acts by promoting blood circulation to prevent blood stasis, by warming the meridians to dissipate cold, and by tonifying qi to nourish the blood. The herbal formulas and single herbs commonly used for the treatment of female infertility are described below. The effects of these herbs on the endocrine regulation effects of the menstrual cycle and the ovulation rate will also be explored. Other commonly prescribed formulas that are used to relieve infertility-related symptoms and diseases such as premenstrual syndrome (Jia-Wei-Xiao-Yao-San), irregular menstrual cycles (Zou-Gui-Wan, You-Gui-Wan), uterine fibroids (Gui-Zhi-Fu-Ling-Wan), diarrhea during menstruation (Shen-Ling-Bai-Zhu-San), dysmenorrhea (Shao-Fu-Zhu-Yu-Tang), abnormal uterine bleeding (Gui-Pi-Tang), amenorrhea, or oligomenorrhea (Si-Wu-Tang), do not fall within the scope of this review.

5.2. Male infertility

A recent study revealed that changes in the metabolic pathways, which regulate aromatic amino acids, tricarboxylic acid cycle, and sphingolipid metabolism may play an important role in the origin of Kidney-Yang deficiency syndrome (KYDS)-associated male infertility [44]. This research offered a new way for metabolomics analysis of seminal plasma to differentiate TCM syndromes of infertile males. The Chinese medicine Huzhangdanshenyin is used for male immune-factor infertility and has been shown to be more effective than prednisone [45]. The medicine works by improving the antisperm-antibody-reversing ratio; and ameliorating sperm indexes such as sperm motility, viability, and density, without severe adverse effects. Another Chinese medicine, Bushen Shengjing Decoction (BSSJD), has the effect of decreasing semen levels of reactive oxygen species (ROS), improving the quality of sperm, and increasing the natural fecundity of patients with severe oligospermia and azoospermia (SOA), thus raising the viability of their sperm in order to increase the ovarian fertilization rate and clinical pregnancy rate in ICSI cycles [46].

5.3. Chinese herbal formulas for infertility

5.3.1. Dang-Gui-Sha-Yao-San

Dang-Gui-Sha-Yao-San consists of Angelicae sinensis Radix, Paeoniae Radix, Poriz, Atractylodis ovatae Rhizoma, Alismatis Rhizoma, and Ligustici Rhizoma. According to the principles of TCM, Dang-Gui-Shao-Yao-San has the effect of nourishing liver blood, invigorating the spleen, and eliminating wetness. A previous study which used a Grading of Recommendations Assessment, Development and Evaluation method (GRADE) to evaluate the quality of evidence for Dang-Gui-Sha-Yao-San concluded that this formula was likely to be beneficial and safe for the treatment of primary dysmenorrhea [47]. Another clinical study showed that it may be useful for resolving the symptoms of mild or moderate hypochromic anemia secondary to uterine myoma-induced menorrhagia [48].

5.3.2. *Wen-Jing-Tang*

Wen-Jing-Tang consists of Cinnamomi Ramulus, Evodiae Fructus, Ligustici Rhizoma, Angelicae sinensis Radix, Paeoniae Radix, Zingiberis Rhizoma Recens, Moutan Radicis Cortex, Ophiopogonis Tuber, Pinelliae Tuber, Ginseng Radix, Glycyrrhizae Radix, and Asini Corii Gelatinum. According to the principles of TCM, Wen-Jing-Tang has the effect of promoting blood circulation to dispel blood stasis, of dispelling cold by warming the meridians, of benefiting qi, and of nourishing the blood. Wen-Jing-Tang has been shown to effectively regulate endocrine conditions such as plasma LH and estradiol levels in PCOS patients with ovulatory dysfunction without taking eight-principle pattern identification into consideration. The study concluded that Wen-Jing-Tang can be used to treat PCOS in women with various constitutions (as determined by the matching theory of eight-principle pattern identification) in clinical management [49]. Another report showed that combined therapy with Wen-Jing-Tang and clomiphene induced ovulation without OHSS in infertile patients who did not respond to clomiphene citrate alone [50].

5.3.3. *Jia-Wei-Xiao-Yao-San*

Jia-Wei-Xiao-Yao-San consists of Moutan Radicis Cortex, Radix Paeoniae Rubra, Bupleuri Radix, Angelicae Sinensis Radix, Atractylodis Ovatae Rhizoma, Poria, Glycyrrhizae Radix, Zingiberis Rhizoma Recens, and Menthae Herba. According to the principles of TCM, Jia-Wei-Xiao-Yao-San disperses stagnated liver qi, suppresses heat, and nourishes the blood. According to the NHIRD in Taiwan, Jia-Wei-Xiao-Yao-San-based Chinese herbal medicine combinations were most frequently used for PMS and primary dysmenorrhea [51]. However, the exact mechanism whereby Jia-Wei-Xiao-Yao-San improves fertility is unclear. In one study, Jia-Wei-Xiao-Yao-San had no effect on serum levels of E2 and FSH, but did improve climacteric symptoms, especially in patients with hormone replacement therapy resistance who strongly complained of psychological symptoms [52]. These findings imply that Jia-Wei-Xiao-Yao-San may affect fertility via as-yet undiscovered mechanisms.

5.3.4. *You-Gui-Wan*

You-Gui-Wan consists of Rhizoma Rehmanniae Praeparata, Rhizoma Dioscoreae, Fructus Lycii, Fructus Corni, Eucommia ulmoides Oliv, Semen Cuscutae, Colla Cornus Cervi, Angelicae sinensis Radix, Radix Aconiti Praeparata, and Cinnamomum cassia Blume. According to the principles of TCM, You-Gui-Wan acts by gently reinforcing the Kidney-Yang, supplementing body essence, and replenishing blood. Previous research has shown that You-Gui-Wan medicated serum can significantly increase the percentage of mature oocytes, and modulate mRNA expression of a number of signaling molecules including protein kinase A (PKA), cAMP-response element binding protein (CREB), mitogen-activated protein kinases (MAPK), protein kinase C (PKC), protein kinase G (PKG), maturation promoting factor (MPF), as well

http://dx.doi.org/10.5772/66971

as concentrations of cyclic adenosine monophosphate (cAMP), cyclic guanosine monophosphate (cGMP), and nitric oxide (NO) [53]. It has also been reported that patients treated with You-Gui-Wan had higher rates of successful IVF compared to those treated with FSH (with or without normal serum). In animal studies, You-Gui-Wan has been shown to increase sperm fertilizing ability by increasing sperm acrosin activity and promoting the acrosome reaction, which resulted in a higher percentage of zygotes in mice treated with You-Gui-Wan compared to control mice [54].

5.3.5. *Zou-Gui-Wan*

Zou-Gui-Wan consists of Colla Cornus Cervi, Colla Plastri Testudinis, Rhizoma Rehmanniae Praeparata, Rhizoma Dioscoreae, Fructus Lycii, Fructus Corni, Radix Cyathulae, and Semen Cuscutae. According to the principles of TCM, You-Gui-Wan gently reinforces the Kidney-Yang, supplements body essence, and replenishes the marrow. Zou-Gui-Wan has also been shown to affect gene expression within germ cells, whereas You-Gui-Wan has stronger effects on estradiol production during the differentiation of stem cells derived from human first trimester umbilical cords into oocyte-like cells *in vitro* [55]. Another report showed that Zou-Gui-Wan promptly and effectively restores ovarian function in patients with POF after failed treatment with clomiphene citrate for 8 months [56].

5.4. Single Chinese herbs for infertility

5.4.1. *Herba Cistanche*

Herba Cistanche, also called Rou Cong Rong in Chinese, originated from Cistanche deserticola Y.C. Ma. According to the principles of TCM, Herba Cistanche invigorates the kidney-yin, and replenishes the vital essence and the blood. It is used as a roborant in a formula for chronic renal disease, impotence, female infertility, morbid leucorrhea, profuse menorrhagia, and senile constipation [57]. It also controls the hypothalamic-pituitary-adrenal (HPA) and HPG axes, which may induce a balanced and smooth sexual energy effect [58]. Herba Cistanche also has aphrodisiac effects and can increase serum levels of progesterone and testosterone, improve sperm count and sperm motility, and decrease the number of abnormal sperm [59].

5.4.2. *Semen Cuscutae*

Semen Cuscutae, also called Tu Si Zi in Chinese, originated from Cuscuta chinensis Lam. According to the principles of TCM, Semen Cuscutae tonifies the kidney and is also believed to arrest spontaneous emission and prevent abortion. It has a multitude of other uses, including antiaging and anti-inflammatory, antiabortifacient, and aphrodisiac, among others [60]. One study has demonstrated that flavonoids obtained from semen cuscutae (FSCs) can be used in the treatment of ovarian endocrine dysfunction in psychologically stressed rats through increasing luteinizing hormone receptor (LHR) expression in the ovaries and estrogen receptor (ER) expression in the hippocampus, hypothalamus, and pituitaries, but without any effect on follicle-stimulating hormone receptor (FSHR) expression in the ovaries [61]. Another study demonstrated that total flavones from semen cuscutae (TFSC) treatment can improve Kidney-Yang deficiency symptoms by recovering the levels of testosterone and increasing androgen receptor (AR) mRNA and protein expression in the testicles and kidneys [62].

5.4.3. Herba Leonuri Japonici

Herba Leonuri Japonici, commonly called Chinese motherwort, originated from Leonurus japonicus Houtt (Labiatae). Related variants of this species include Leonurus sibiricus auct. pl., Leonurus artemisia (Lour.) S.Y. Hu., Leonurus heterophyllus sweet, and Stachys artemisia Lour [63]. According to the principles of TCM, Herba Leonuri Japonici promotes blood flow to regulate menstruation and induces diuresis to alleviate edema. It is also referred to as Yi Mu Cao in Chinese, which translates literally into "beneficial herb for mothers," and is used to manage dysmenorrhea, amenorrhea, menoxenia, lochia, edema, and other gynecological problems but is contraindicated in pregnancy due to the possibility of stimulating the uterus [63]. The aqueous extract from the aerial part of Leonurus artemisia has the potential to treat dysmenorrhea by increasing the serum progesterone level, inhibiting inflammation, relaxing uterine spasms, and decreasing prostaglandin F2α (PGF2α) and prostaglandin E2 (PGE2) concentrations in uterine smooth muscle [64].

6. Acupuncture and moxibustion

As with TCM and single Chinese herbal therapy, acupuncture and moxibustion have also been used to treat female or male infertility for hundreds of years. Traditionally, acupuncture and moxibustion were performed by inserting needles or burning moxa sticks into specific points (acupoints) on the meridians. Acupuncture and moxibustion work by regulating energy flow, also called Qi in Chinese, over the meridians. Newer therapeutic methods include electro-acupuncture (EA), laser-acupuncture, burning moxa granules on the top of the needles, points pasting, and far-infrared moxibustion. Some meridians or acupoints have been indicated for the management of gynecological or obstetric problems, and these include Taichong (LR 3), Taixi (KI 3), Sanyinchiao (SP 6), and Gongsun (SP 4). These points were the earliest recorded in the Chinese classic Huangdi Neijing (the Classic of Inner Canon of Huangdi) around the time of the Han dynasty, and in the Chinese classic Zhenjiu Jiayi Jing (the A-B Classic of Acupuncture and Moxibustion) during the Jin dynasty.

6.1. Male infertility

Gonadotropin-releasing hormone (GnRH) is released by the hypothalamus and stimulates ovulation and sperm production in women and men, respectively. Thus, its deficiency contributes to both male and female infertility [65]. One study showed that repeated EA on the arcuate nucleus (Arc) can regulate the function of the HPG axis by suppressing Arc discharge, serum testosterone, sperm count, and GnRH mRNA expression [66]. Therefore, electrical stimulation may be an effective alternative to medications to regulate the HPG axis [67]. Another clinical trial in humans showed that 10-Hz EA stimulation of the abdominal acupuncture points ST-29 (guilai) increased testicular blood flow (TBF), but simple needle insertion and 2-Hz EA stimulation did not [68]. The combination of acupuncture and moxibustion treatment has also been shown to increase the percentage of normal-form sperm in infertile patients with oligoastenoteratozoospermia in a prospective, controlled, and blinded study, but the mechanisms remain unknown [69]. Another study revealed that acupuncture can improve

http://dx.doi.org/10.5772/66971

quick sperm motility, increase the normal sperm ratio, and improve fertilization rates and embryo quality in cases of idiopathic male infertility with failed ICSI [70]. According to the results of a systemic review from China regarding the treatment of male infertility, acupuncture appears to be as effective as TCM and more effective than western medicine alone, and its ability to improve sperm concentration and increase the level of grade a pulse b sperm is increased when applied together with either TCM or western medicine [71].

6.2. Female infertility

There is evidence to suggest that acupuncture stimulation of acupoints of the conception vessel, spleen, kidney, and bladder meridians improves clinical symptoms in patients with diminished ovarian reserve (DOR), and also lowers serum FSH, LH, and estradiol [E(2)] levels through regulation of the hypothalamic-pituitary-ovarian (HPO) axis [72]. A randomized, prospective, controlled clinical study revealed that acupuncture during the luteal phase of IVF/ICSI cycles increased clinical pregnancy and ongoing pregnancy rates [73]. Acupuncture improves IVF outcomes through four potential mechanisms: (1) by increasing blood flow to the uterus; (2) by regulating neuroendocrinological factors and the ovaries; (3) by modulating cytokine levels; and (4) by decreasing levels of anxiety, stress, and depression [74]. A successful pregnancy relies on the presence of adequate uterine blood flow and endometrial thickness, and these factors are especially important in pregnancies conceived through IVF and ET [67]. A study of infertile women with a high pulsatility index (PI) and downregulated with a GnRH analog to exclude any fluctuating endogenous hormone effects on the PI, revealed that EA reduced uterine artery blood flow impedance [75]. However, the literature on the efficacy of acupuncture treatment for endometriosis, immune and pelvic inflammatory disease-related infertility or subfertility is sparse. One study on women with steroid-induced polycystic ovaries demonstrated that EA modulates the neuroendocrinological state of the ovaries by inhibiting endothelin-1 and nerve growth factor (NGF), and NGF mRNA expression, most likely by modulating sympathetic activity in the ovaries [76]. Another similar study on estradiol valerate-induced polycystic ovaries demonstrated that EA treatments change the neuroendocrinological state in the ovaries by suppressing corticotropin-releasing factor, which may play an important role in reproductive failure [77]. Finally, the results of the Fertility Problem Inventory (FPI) and Beck Anxiety Inventory (BAI) questionnaires revealed that women suffer greater anxiety and sexual infertility stress than men [78]. High levels of stress affect female hormone levels and disrupt ovulation by affecting the HPO axis [67]. These studies all highlight a need for additional research into the potential benefits of acupuncture and moxibustion for the management of infertile patients.

7. Conclusions

Infertility results in a country with a low birth rate and an aging population, and thus there is vested interest in treating this problem by using both complementary and alternative therapies, in addition to conventional western medicine. There is increasing scientific evidence to support a role for TCM in the management of male and female infertility, but further studies are needed to elucidate the efficacy of this alternative therapy.

Abbreviations

AI	artificial insemination
AMH	anti-Müllerian hormone
AR	androgen receptor
ART	assisted reproductive technology
BAI	Beck Anxiety Inventory
BMI	body mass index
BSSJD	Bushen Shengjing Decoction
cAMP	concentrations of cyclic adenosine monophosphate
CCCT	the clomiphene citrate challenge test
cGMP	cyclic guanosine monophosphate
CREB	cAMP-response element binding protein
DOR	diminished ovarian reserve
E2	estradiol
EA	electro-acupuncture
ER	estrogen receptor
FPI	Fertility Problem Inventory
FSCs	flavonoids from Semen cuscutaes
FSH	follicle-stimulating hormone
FSHR	follicle-stimulating hormone receptor
GnRH	gonadotropin-releasing hormone
GnRHa	gonadotrophin-releasing hormone analogue
GRADE	Grading of Recommendations Assessment, Development and Evaluation
HBV/HCV	hepatitis B/C virus
hCG	human chorionic gonadotropin
HIV	human immunodeficiency virus
HPG	hypothalamic-pituitary-gonad
ICSI	intracytoplasmic sperm injection
IUI	intra-uterine insemination
IVF-ET	*in vitro* fertilization and embryo transfer
KYDS	Kidney-Yang deficiency syndrome
LH	luteinizing hormone
LHR	luteinizing hormone receptor
MAPK	mitogen-activated protein kinases
MPF	maturation-promoting factor

http://dx.doi.org/10.5772/66971

mRNA	messenger ribonucleic acid
NGF	nerve growth factor
NHIRD	National Health Insurance Research Database
NO	nitric oxide
OCs	oral contraceptives
OH	ovarian hyperstimulation
OHSS	ovarian hyperstimulation syndrome
Pap	Papanicolaou
PCOS	polycystic ovary syndrome
PGE2	prostaglandin E2
PGF2α	prostaglandin F2α
PHA	hypothalamic-pituitary-adrenal
PKA	protein kinase A
PKC	protein kinase C
PKG	protein kinase G
PMS	premenstrual syndrome
POF	premature ovarian failure
ROS	reactive oxygen species
SOA	oligospermatism and azoospermia
TBF	testicular blood flow
TCM	traditional Chinese medicine
TFSC	total flavones from Semen cuscutae
TI	timed intercourse
WHO	World Health Organization

Author details

Yen-Nung Liao[1], Wen-Long Hu[1, 2, 3] and Yu-Chiang Hung[1, 4*]

*Address all correspondence to: hungyuchiang@gmail.com

1 Department of Chinese Medicine, Kaohsiung Chang Gung Memorial Hospital and School of Traditional Chinese Medicine, Chang Gung University College of Medicine, Kaohsiung, Taiwan

2 Kaohsiung Medical University College of Medicine, Kaohsiung, Taiwan

3 Fooyin University College of Nursing, Kaohsiung, Taiwan

4 School of Chinese Medicine for Post Baccalaureate, I-Shou University, Kaohsiung, Taiwan

References

[1] The ESHRE (European Society for Human Reproduction and Embryology) Capri Workshop. Infertility revisited: the state of the art today and tomorrow. Hum Reprod. 1996;11:1779–1807.

[2] Bhattacharya S, Johnson N, Tijani HA, Hart R, Pandey S, Gibreel AF. Female infertility. BMJ Clin Evid. 2010; 2010:pii: 0819.

[3] Kuohung W, Hornstein MD. Introduction of Infertility [Internet]. 2016. Available from: http://www.uptodate.com/contents/evaluation-of-female-infertility?source=search_result&search=infertility&selectedTitle=2%7E150. [Accessed: 2016-06-30]

[4] Mascarenhas MN, Flaxman SR, Boerma T. Vanderpoel S, Stevens GA. National, regional, and global trends in infertility prevalence since 1990: a systematic analysis of 277 health surveys. PLoS Med. 2012;9:e1001356. DOI: 10.1371/journal.pmed.1001356

[5] Chandra A, Copen CE, Stephen EH. Infertility and impaired fecundity in the United States, 1982-2010: data from the National Survey of Family Growth. Natl Health Stat Report. 2013;67:1–18, 1 p following 19.

[6] Taiwan. Department of Household Registration Affairs, Ministry of Interior. Fertility Rates of Childbearing Age Women [Internet]. 2016. Available from: http://sowf.moi.gov.tw/stat/year/y02-04.xls. [Accessed: 2016-07-25]

[7] Meng QQ, Zhang YL, Ren AG. Infertility rate in married couples of reproductive age in China: a systematic review and meta-analysis. Zhonghua Liu Xing Bing Xue Za Zhi. 2013;34:826–831. DOI: 10.3760/cmad.issn.0254-6450.2013.08.017

[8] Rutstein SO, Shah IH. Infecundity, infertility, and childlessness in developing countries. DHS Comparative Reports No. 9. Calverton, MD: ORC Macro and the World Health Organization. 2004.

[9] Taiwan. The Executive Yuan of the Republic of China (Taiwan). POPULATION POLICY WHITE PAPER-Fewer Children, Population Aging and Immigration. Taipei. 2013. p. 5–14.

[10] Stellar C, Garcia-Moreno C, Temmerman M, van der Poel S. A systematic review and narrative report of the relationship between infertility, subfertility, and intimate partner violence. Int J Gynaecol Obstet. 2016;133:3–8. DOI: 10.1016/j.ijgo.2015.08.012

[11] Gadducci A, Guerrieri ME, Genazzani AR. Fertility drug use and risk of ovarian tumors: a debated clinical challenge. Gynecol Endocrinol. 2013;29:30–35. DOI: 10.3109/09513590.2012.705382

[12] Riskin-Mashiah S. Infertility, fertility treatment and breast cancer risk. Harefuah. 2013;152:600–604, 623.

[13] Armstrong S, Akande V. What is the best treatment option for infertile women aged 40 and over? J Assist Reprod Genet. 2013;30:667–671. DOI: 10.1007/s10815-013-9980-6

[14] Verkuijlen J, Verhaak C, Nelen WL, Wilkinson J, Farquhar C. Psychological and educational interventions for subfertile men and women. Cochrane Database Syst Rev. 2016;3:CD011034. DOI: 10.1002/14651858.CD011034.pub2

[15] Anawalt BD. Approach to male infertility and induction of spermatogenesis. J Clin Endocrinol Metab. 2013;98:3532–3542. DOI: 10.1210/jc.2012-2400

[16] Kuohung W, Hornstein MD. Overview of infertility [Internet]. 2016. Available from: http://www.uptodate.com/contents/causes-of-female-infertility?source=machineLearning&search=infertility&selectedTitle=4%7E150&sectionRank=5&anchor=H16#H16. [Accessed: 2016-07-25]

[17] Sharlip ID, Jarow JP, Belker AM, Lipshultz LI, Sigman M, Thomas AJ, Schlegel PN, Howards SS, Nehra A, Damewood MD, Overstreet JW, Sadovsky R. Best practice policies for male infertility. Fertil Steril. 2002;77:873–882.

[18] Lee LK, Foo KY. Recent insights on the significance of transcriptomic and metabolomic analysis of male factor infertility. Clin Biochem. 2014;47:973–982. DOI: 10.1016/j.clinbiochem.2014.05.053

[19] Yang M, He Y, Huang L, et al. Epidemiological investigation of constitution of sterility patients. J New Chin Med. 2010;42:55–56.

[20] Case AM. Infertility evaluation and management. Strategies for family physicians. Can Fam Physician. 2003;49:1465–1472.

[21] Crawford NM, Steiner AZ. Age-related infertility. Obstet Gynecol Clin North Am. 2015;42:15–25. DOI: 10.1016/j.ogc.2014.09.005

[22] Stoop D, Cobo A, Silber S. Fertility preservation for age-related fertility decline. Lancet. 2014;384:1311–1319. DOI: 10.1016/S0140-6736(14)61261-7

[23] Ecklund LC, Usadi RS. Endocrine and reproductive effects of polycystic ovarian syndrome. Obstet Gynecol Clin North Am. 2015;42:55–65. DOI: 10.1016/j.ogc.2014.09.003

[24] Legendre G, Catala L, Morinière C, Lacoeuille C, Boussion F, Sentilhes L, Descamps P. Relationship between ovarian cysts and infertility: what surgery and when? Fertil Steril. 2014;101:608–614. DOI: 10.1016/j.fertnstert.2014.01.021

[25] Kodaman PH. Current strategies for endometriosis management. Obstet Gynecol Clin North Am. 2015;42:87–101. DOI: 10.1016/j.ogc.2014.10.005

[26] Al-Jabri S, Tulandi T. Management and prevention of pelvic adhesions. Semin Reprod Med. 2011;29:130–137. DOI: 10.1055/s-0031-1272475

[27] Hamilton CJ, Evers JL, Hoogland HJ. Ovulatory disorders and inflammatory adnexal damage: a neglected cause of the failure of fertility microsurgery. Br J Obstet Gynaecol. 1986;93:282–284.

[28] Franklin RR. Reduction of ovarian adhesions by the use of Interceed. Ovarian Adhesion Study Group. Obstet Gynecol. 1995;86:335–340. PMID: 7651638

[29] Chen B, Yang C, Sahebally Z, Jin H. Unilateral ovarian and fallopian tube agenesis in an infertile patient with a normal uterus. Exp Ther Med. 2014;8:831–835. DOI: 10.3892/etm.2014.1825

[30] Narayanan R, Rajeev MA. Duplication of the fallopian tube. J Hum Reprod Sci. 2008;1:35–36. PMID: 19562063 PMCID: PMC2700681

[31] Briceag I, Costache A, Purcarea VL, Cergan R, Dumitru M, Briceag I, Sajin M, Ispas AT. Fallopian tubes—literature review of anatomy and etiology in female infertility. J Med Life. 2015;8:129–131. PMID: 25866566 PMCID: PMC4392087

[32] Mah PM, Webster J. Hyperprolactinemia: etiology, diagnosis, and management. Semin Reprod Med. 2002;20:365–374. DOI: 10.1055/s-2002-36709

[33] Naumburg EH. Chapter 1: Interview and The Health History. In: Bickley LS, Hoekelman RA editors. Bate's Guide to Physocal Examination and History Taking. 7th ed. Philadelphia: Lippincott Williams & Wilkins; 1999. p. 35–39.

[34] Adam HB, Howard SJ. Alan HD. Chapter 4: Investing Infertility. Infertility in Practice. 1st ed. New York: Churchill Livingstone; 1997. pp. 49–54.

[35] Wendy K, Mark DH. [Internet]. 2016. Available from: http://www.uptodate.com/contents/evaluation-of-female-infertility?source=search_result&search=infertility+evaluation&selectedTitle=1%7E150#H3 [Accessed: 2016-10-10]

[36] Bickely LS, Hoekelman RA editors. Chapter 12: Male Genitalia and Hernias. Bate's Guide to Physocal Examination and History Taking. 7th ed. Philadelphia: Lippincott Williams & Wilkins; 1999. pp. 387–403.

[37] Ozgur K, Humaidan P, Coetzee K. Segmented ART—the new era in ART? Reprod Biol. 2016;16:91–103. DOI: 10.1016/j.repbio.2016.04.001

[38] Farquhar C, Rishworth JR, Brown J, Nelen WL, Marjoribanks J. Assisted reproductive technology: an overview of Cochrane reviews. Cochrane Database Syst Rev. 2015;7:CD010537. DOI: 10.1002/14651858.CD010537.pub4

[39] Veltman-Verhulst SM, Hughes E, Ayeleke RO, Cohlen BJ. Intra-uterine insemination for unexplained subfertility. Cochrane Database Syst Rev. 2016;2:CD001838. DOI: 10.1002/14651858.CD001838.pub5

[40] Ginsburg ES. Procedure for Intrauterine Insemination (IUI) using Processed Sperm [Internet]. 2016. Available from: http://www.uptodate.com/contents/procedure-for-intrauterine-insemination-iui-using-processed-sperm?source=search_result&search=Intrauterine+insemination+for+unexplained+subfertility+UPTODATE&selectedTitle=2%7E150. [Accessed: 2016-07-27]

[41] Ried K, Stuart K. Efficacy of traditional Chinese herbal medicine in the management of female infertility: a systematic review. Complement Ther Med. 2011;19:319–331. DOI: 10.1016/j.ctim.2011.09.003

[42] Zhu S, Liu D, Huang W, Wang Q, Wang Q, Zhou L, Feng G. Post-laparoscopic oral contraceptive combined with Chinese herbal mixture in treatment of infertility and pain associated with minimal or mild endometriosis: a randomized controlled trial. BMC Complement Altern Med. 2014;14:222. DOI: 10.1186/1472-6882-14-222

[43] Hung YC, Kao CW, Lin CC, Liao YN, Wu BY, Hung IL, Hu WL. Chinese herbal products for female infertility in Taiwan: a population-based cohort study. Medicine. 2016;9511:e3075. DOI: 10.1097/MD.0000000000003075

[44] Chen X, Hu C, Dai J, Chen L. Metabolomics analysis of seminal plasma in infertile males with kidney-yang deficiency: a preliminary study. Evid Based Complement Alternat Med. 2015;2015:892930. DOI: 10.1155/2015/892930

[45] Lu TK, Ouyang HG, Jin GY, Hong YS, Zou Q, Lin ZY, Deng LS, Guo YB. Clinical study on the treatment of male immune infertility by Huzhangdanshenyin. Zhonghua Nan Ke Xue. 2006;12:750–755. DOI :10.13263/j .cnki .nja.2006.08.026

[46] Zhang HQ, Zhao HX, Zhang AJ. Male infertility with severe oligospermatism and azoospermia treated by Bushen Shengjing Decoction combined with intracytoplasmic sperm injection. Zhongguo Zhong Xi Yi Jie He Za Zhi. 2007;27:972–975.

[47] Latthe PM, Champaneria R, Khan KS. Dysmenorrhoea. BMJ Clin Evid. 2011;2011:pii: 0813.

[48] Akase T, Akase T, Onodera S, Jobo T, Matsushita R, Kaneko M, Tashiro S. A comparative study of the usefulness of toki-shakuyaku-san and an oral iron preparation in the treatment of hypochromic anemia in cases of uterine myoma. Yakugaku Zasshi. 2003;123:817–824.

[49] Ushiroyama T, Hosotani T, Mori K, Yamashita Y, Ikeda A, Ueki M. Effects of switching to wen-jing-tang (unkei-to) from preceding herbal preparations selected by eight-principle pattern identification on endocrinological status and ovulatory induction in women with polycystic ovary syndrome. Am J Chin Med. 2006;34:177–187. DOI: 10.1142/S0192415X06003746

[50] Yoshimoto Y, Miyake A, Tasaka K, Aono T, Tanizawa O. Ovulation following combined therapy with wen-jing-tang and clomiphene citrate therapy in anovulatory women. Am J Chin Med. 1989;17:243–244. DOI: 10.1142/S0192415X89000334

[51] Chen HY, Huang BS, Lin YH, Su IH, Yang SH, Chen JL, Huang JW, Chen YC. Identifying Chinese herbal medicine for premenstrual syndrome: implications from a nationwide database. BMC Complement Altern Med. 2014;14:206. DOI: 10.1186/1472-6882-14-206

[52] Hidaka T, Yonezawa R, Saito S. Kami-shoyo-san, Kampo (Japanese traditional medicine), is effective for climacteric syndrome, especially in hormone-replacement-therapy-resistant patients who strongly complain of psychological symptoms. J Obstet Gynaecol Res. 2013;39:223–228. DOI: 10.1111/j.1447-0756.2012.01936.x

[53] Jiang XH, Deng YL, Lu H, Duan H, Zhen X, Hu X, Liang X, Yie SM. Effect of rat medicated serum containing you gui wan on mouse oocyte in vitro maturation and subsequent fertilization competence. Evid Based Complement Alternat Med. 2014;2014:152010. DOI: 10.1155/2014/152010

[54] Jiang XH, Yie SM, Zhen X, Den YL, Liang X, Hu X, Li LM, Li QJ, Cao S, Lu H. Effect of You Gui Wan on mouse sperm fertilising ability in vivo and in vitro. Andrologia. 2014;46:283–289. DOI: 10.1111/and.12075

[55] Hu X, Lu H, Deng YL, Wan Q, Yie SM. Effect of rat medicated serum containing Zuo Gui Wan and/or You Gui Wan on the differentiation of stem cells derived from human first trimester umbilical cord into oocyte-like cells in vitro. Evid Based Complement Alternat Med. 2015;2015:825805. DOI: 10.1155/2015/825805

[56] Chao SL, Huang LW, Yen HR. Pregnancy in premature ovarian failure after therapy using Chinese herbal medicine. Chang Gung Med J. 2003;26:449–452.

[57] Li Z, Lin H, Gu L, Gao J, Tzeng CM. Herba Cistanche (Rou Cong-Rong): one of the best pharmaceutical gifts of traditional Chinese medicine. Front Pharmacol. 2016;7:41. DOI: 10.3389/fphar.2016.00041

[58] Li Z, Lin H, Gu L, Gao J, Tzeng CM. Supplementary material of Herba Cistanche (Rou Cong-Rong): one of the best pharmaceutical gifts of traditional Chinese medicine. Front Pharmacol [Internet]. 2016. Available from: http://journal.frontiersin.org/article/10.3389/fphar.2016.00041. [Accessed: 2016-07-27]

[59] Wang T, Chen C, Yang M, Deng B, Kirby GM, Zhang X. Cistanche tubulosa ethanol extract mediates rat sex hormone levels by induction of testicular steroidgenic enzymes. Pharm Biol. 2016;54:481–487. DOI: 10.3109/13880209.2015.1050114

[60] Donnapee S, Li J, Yang X, Ge AH, Donkor PO, Gao XM, Chang YX. Cuscuta chinensis Lam.: a systematic review on ethnopharmacology, phytochemistry and pharmacology of an important traditional herbal medicine. J Ethnopharmacol. 2014;157:292–308. DOI: 10.1016/j.jep.2014.09.032

[61] Ke J, Duan R. Effects of flavonoids from semen cuscutae on the hippocampal-hypothalamic-pituitary-ovarian sex hormone receptors in female rats exposed to psychological stress. Clin Exp Obstet Gynecol. 2013;40:271–274.

[62] Yang J, Wang Y, Bao Y, Guo J. The total flavones from Semen cuscutae reverse the reduction of testosterone level and the expression of androgen receptor gene in kidney-yang deficient mice. J Ethnopharmacol. 2008;119:166–171. DOI: 10.1016/j.jep.2008.06.027

[63] Shang X, Pan H, Wang X, He H, Li M. Leonurus japonicus Houtt.: ethnopharmacology, phytochemistry and pharmacology of an important traditional Chinese medicine. J Ethnopharmacol. 2014;152:14–32. DOI: 10.1016/j.jep.2013.12.052

[64] Jin RM, Chen ZS, Chen CX. Effects of motherwort on dysmenorrhea. Chin J Mod Appl Pharm. 2004;21:90–93. DOI :10.13748/j .cnki .issn1007-7693.2004.02.003

[65] Messinis IE. Ovarian feedback, mechanism of action and possible clinical implications. Hum Reprod Update. 2006;12:557–571. DOI: 10.1093/humupd/dml020

[66] Zhaohui Z, Yugui C, Yuanming Z, Xuesong W, Xiaobing J, Zhice X, Guipeng D, Qianle T, Yue J. Effect of acupuncture on pubertal development of rats and rabbits at different developmental stages. Neuropeptides. 2007;41:249–261. DOI: 10.1016/j.npep.2007.02.003

[67] Xia JF, Inagaki Y, Zhang JF, Wang L, Song PP. Chinese medicine as complementary therapy for female infertility. Chin J Integr Med, 2016;Epub ahead of print. DOI: 10.1007/s11655-016-2510-5

[68] Cakmak YO, Akpinar IN, Ekinci G, Bekiroglu N. Point- and frequency-specific response of the testicular artery to abdominal electroacupuncture in humans. Fertil Steril. 2008;90:1732–1738. DOI: 10.1016/j.fertnstert.2007.08.013

[69] Gurfinkel E, Cedenho AP, Yamamura Y, Srougi M. Effects of acupuncture and moxa treatment in patients with semen abnormalities. Asian J Androl. 2003;5:345–348.

[70] Zhang M, Huang G, Lu F, Paulus WE, Sterzik K. Influence of acupuncture on idiopathic male infertility in assisted reproductive technology. J Huazhong Univ Sci Technol Med Sci. 2002;22:228–230.

[71] He Y, Chen CT, Qian LH, Xia CL, Li J, Li SQ, Liu BP. Acupuncture treatment of male infertility: a systematic review. Zhonghua Nan Ke Xue. 2015;21:637–645. DOI: 10.13263/j.cnki.nja.2015.07.012

[72] Tang WL, Hu YH, He XH. Acupuncture stimulation of acupoints of multiple Meridians for patients with diminished ovarian reserve of both Yin and Yang deficiency. Zhen Ci Yan Jiu. 2015;40:479–483, 488. DOI: 10.13702/j.1000-0607.2015.06.010

[73] Dieterle S, Ying G, Hatzmann W, Neuer A. Effect of acupuncture on the outcome of in vitro fertilization and intracytoplasmic sperm injection: a randomized, prospective, controlled clinical study. Fertil Steril. 2006;85:1347–1351. DOI: 10.1016/j.fertnstert.2005.09.062

[74] Anderson BJ, Haimovici F, Ginsburg ES, Schust DJ, Wayne PM. In vitro fertilization and acupuncture: clinical efficacy and mechanistic basis. Altern Ther Health Med. 2007;13:38–48.

[75] Stener-Victorin E, Waldenström U, Andersson SA, Wikland M. Reduction of blood flow impedance in the uterine arteries of infertile women with electro-acupuncture. Hum Reprod. 1996;11:1314–1317.

[76] Stener-Victorin E, Lundeberg T, Cajander S, Aloe L, Manni L, Waldenström U, Janson PO. Steroid-induced polycystic ovaries in rats: effect of electro-acupuncture on concentrations of endothelin-1 and nerve growth factor (NGF), and expression of NGF mRNA in the ovaries, the adrenal glands, and the central nervous system. Reprod Biol Endocrinol. 2003;1:33.

[77] Stener-Victorin E, Lundeberg T, Waldenström U, Bileviciute-Ljungar I, Janson PO. Effects of electro-acupuncture on corticotropin-releasing factor in rats with experimentally-induced polycystic ovaries. Neuropeptides. 2001;35:227–231. DOI: 10.1054/npep.2002.0878

[78] Peterson BD, Newton CR, Feingold T. Anxiety and sexual stress in men and women undergoing infertility treatment. Fertil Steril. 2007;88:911–914. DOI: 10.1016/j.fertnstert.2006.12.023

Chapter 6

Clearance of Free Silica in Rat Lungs by Spraying with Chinese Herbal Kombucha

Sheng-jun Jiang, Nai-fang Fu, Zhi-chao Dong, Chang-hui Luo, Jun-cai Wu, Yan-yan Zheng, Yong-jin Gan, Jian-an Ling, Heng-qiu Liang, Dan-yu Liang, Jing Xie, Xiao-qin Chen, Xian-jun Li, Rui-hui Pan, Zuo-Xing Chen and Lu-lu Zhang

Additional information is available at the end of the chapter

http://dx.doi.org/10.5772/66970

Abstract

The effects of spraying with kombucha and Chinese herbal kombucha were compared with treatments with tetrandrine in a rat silicosis model. Silica dust (50 mg) was injected into the lungs of rats, which were then treated with one of the experimental treatments for a month. The rats were then killed, and the effects of the treatments were evaluated by examining the extent and severity of the histopathological lesions in the animals' lungs, measuring their organ coefficients and lung collagen contents, determining the dry and wet weights of their lungs, and measuring the free silica content of the dried lungs. In addition, lavage was performed on whole lungs taken from selected rats, and the numbers and types of cells in the lavage fluid were counted. The most effective treatment in terms of the ability to reduce lung collagen content and minimize the formation of pulmonary histopathological lesions was tetrandrine treatment, followed by Chinese herbal kombucha and non-Chinese herbal kombucha. However, the lavage fluid cell counts indicated that tetrandrine treatment had severe adverse effects on macrophage viability. This effect was much less pronounced for the kombucha and Chinese herbal kombucha treatments. Moreover, the free silica levels in the lungs of animals treated with Chinese herbal kombucha were significantly lower than those for any other silica-exposed group. These preliminary results indicate that spraying with Chinese herbal kombucha preparations can effectively promote the discharge of silica dust from lung tissues. Chinese herbal kombucha inhalation may thus be a useful new treatment for silicosis and other pneumoconiosis diseases.

Keywords: clearance, silica particles, rat, silicosis, Chinese herbal kombucha

1. Introduction

Silicosis is a pneumoconiosis disease caused by exposure to various forms of silica dust including crystalline silica and amorphous silica dust [1]. It is caused by the inhalation of fine silica particles, which are deposited in the lungs and ingested by macrophages. This triggers an immune response that stimulates the production of collagen around the particle, resulting in the formation of nodular lesions that obstruct the airways. Occupational exposure to silica dust and the resulting health problems are major public health issues in both developed and developing countries [2]. It was recently reported that 23 million workers in China have been exposed to crystalline silica dust, and that more than ten million workers in India are at risk of exposure [3, 4]. Similarly, more than 1.7 million workers in the USA and more than 3 million workers in Europe are likely to have been exposed to silica dust in the workplace [5, 6]. Silicosis has a range of adverse effects on health, including an increased susceptibility to tuberculosis, lung cancer, and pulmonary heart disease. These problems are exacerbated by the lack of an effective treatment for the condition.

Kombucha is a drink made by fermenting sugar and tea extracts with kombucha. It is rich in acetic acid bacteria, yeast probiotics, acetic acid, and other organic acids that are beneficial to human health and can inhibit the growth of harmful bacteria. It has proven to be a good treatment for atrophic gastritis and gastric ulcer disease and can also help to regulate blood pressure and slow aging and to prevent and treat various diseases [7]. Kombucha contains two notable groups of microorganisms: *Gluconoacetobacter xylinus* (Xylinum) and yeasts. Xylinum secretes bacterial cellulose through holes in its cell walls. Interestingly, kombucha cultures produce bacterial cellulose more efficiently than cultures of Xylinum alone [8, 9]. The bacterial cellulose produced by Kampuchea cultures has a number of properties that make it potentially useful in medical applications, including good biocompatibility, thinness (the cellulose sheets are typically only 0.1 μm thick), and a high-specific surface area. These properties mean that it functions as a nanoscale functional material with a defined three-dimensional structure and a large number of surface-exposed hydroxyl groups, which allow it to form strong noncovalent bonds with water and also a wide range of ions and organic compounds [10]. It has been demonstrated that bacterial cellulose efficiently adsorbs numerous toxic heavy metal ions, including Cu^{2+}, Pb2+, Hg^{2+}, and Cd^{2+}. In addition, it adsorbs a range of nonmetallic toxins such as histamines, ammonia, and NO_2^- and formaldehyde [11–16]. We therefore hypothesized that if kombucha was sprayed into lung tissues, the bacterial cellulose produced by the culture might adsorb dust and protein precipitates that would otherwise cause the symptoms of silicosis.

Chinese herbal kombucha preparations can be made by fermenting extracts of various plants with a Kampuchea culture. If the plants used in these preparations contain biologically active substances, the resulting Chinese herbal kombucha may combine the beneficial effects of the Kampuchea itself with those of the plants. A range of plants and herbs can be used for this purpose, including licorice, *Siratia grosvenori*, mangosteen, and chrysanthemum. Licorice is known to have numerous pharmacological effects and is widely used in traditional medicine. It contains a range of biologically active compounds, including glycyrrhizin, glycyrrhetinic acid, and the licorice flavonoids. Both licorice and the isolated active compounds are known to have antitussive and expectorant properties. Moreover, it is effective against asthma and offers protection against respiratory pathogens [17, 18]. *Siratia grosvenori* is a specific Chinese plant belonging to the family Cucurbitaceae. When dried, its fruit is very sweet and has a cooling effect. It is an important ingredient of "cooling drinks" and is considered to be beneficial for relieving conditions characterized by high body temperatures, such as inflammation. It is used in traditional Chinese medicine to treat chest pains, dry coughs, sore throats, and aphonia [19]. Mangosteen aqueous extracts have been shown to significantly reduce the frequency of coughing in guinea pigs treated with citric acid or capsaicin and inhibits coughing caused by mechanical stimulation [20]. Chrysanthemum is an important medicinal plant that has various pharmacological effects. Among other things, it functions as an antibacterial, anti-inflammatory, vasodilatory, and antitumor agent, as well as reducing blood pressure and acting as an antioxidant [21]. Teas made from the buds of the camellia plant contain many bioactive compounds, including polyphenols, tea polysaccharides, alkaloids, vitamins, and amino acids, as well as various essential metal ions. As a result, they have a wide range of pharmacological activities, including anti-inflammatory, antioxidant, and antithrombosis effects, as well as being useful in the treatment of diabetes and for reducing blood pressure [22, 23].

In light of these facts, we sought to investigate the utility of kombucha and various Chinese herbal Kampuchea mixtures for the treatment of silicosis and other diseases arising from the presence of dust in the lungs. To this end, rats were exposed to silica dust via tracheal injection and then sprayed with Chinese herbal and non-Chinese herbal kombucha solutions. The results of the kombucha treatments were compared to those observed following treatment with tetrandrine, a compound that is known to be useful for mitigating the symptoms of silicosis [24]. The different treatments were evaluated in terms of their effects on lung anatomy, collagen levels in the lung tissues of the experimental animals, and toxicity.

2. Materials and methods

2.1. Materials

Silica dust (99% particle diameter 0.5–10 μm with 80% of particles having diameters of 1–5 μm) was purchased from Sigma-Aldrich. Tetrandrine was purchased from the Zhejiang Zhongyi Pharmaceutical Co., Ltd. A kit for measuring collagen (hydroxyproline) levels was purchased from the Nanjing Jiancheng Bioengineering Institute.

2.2. Preparation of the Kombucha mixtures

Kampuchea strains were purchased from the Beijing Institute of Food Research. A kombucha stock solution was prepared according to the method of Ai-jun Lv [23]. The Chinese herbal extract was prepared by mixing tea (0.2% w/w), licorice (0.5% w/w), dried *Siratia grosvenori* fruit (0.5% w/w), and wild chrysanthemum (0.2% w/w) in water and boiling the resulting mixtures for 20 min. The boiled solution was then filtered, cooled to below 30°C, and mixed with a 20% dilution of the kombucha stock solution. After fermenting at 30°C for 2 weeks, the Chinese herbal kombucha solution was considered ready for use in experiments.

2.3. Experimental animals

Test animals were provided by the Hunan Slack Jingda experimental animal company (License number SCXK; Hunan). The animals used were specific pathogen-free (SPF) Sprague-Dawley (SD) rats that had been held under quarantine for 5 days.

2.4. Tracheal injection of method for the contamination of silica dust

A 50 mg/mL standard suspension of quartz (silica) dust in saline was prepared [25–27]. Prior to tracheal injection, samples of the stock solution were autoclaved and then mixed with mycillin (4000 U/mL). The experimental animals were then anaesthetized under sterile conditions and subjected to intratracheal injection with 1 mL of the sterile mycillin-containing silica dust suspension in lungs.

2.5. Experimental groups and treatments

The 150 experimental animals weighed 180–220 g each and were randomly allocated to five different groups of 30 animals each, 15 males and 15 females (see **Table 1**).

Group	Treatment
Chinese herbal kombucha treatment group	Starting 4 days after being injected with silica, the rats were sprayed with Chinese herbal kombucha. Each rat was sprayed 20 times in the morning and 20 times in the afternoon for 5 consecutive days per week, over a 4-week period
Kombucha treatment group	Starting 4 days after being injected with silica, the rats were sprayed with non-Chinese herbal kombucha. Each rat was sprayed 20 times in the morning and in the afternoon for 5 consecutive days per week, over a 4-week period
Tetrandrine treatment group	The rats were treated with tetrandrine by lavage. Each rat was dosed with 15 mg three times per week for 4 weeks
Positive control group	Starting 4 days after being injected with silica, the rats were sprayed with a 1 g/L solution of NaCl. Each rat was sprayed 20 times in the morning and 20 times in the afternoon for 5 consecutive days per week, over a 4-week period
Negative control group	Synchronously operated with the positive control group, at the fourth day of instilled with silica. Each rat was sprayed 20 times continuously once in the morning and once in the afternoon for 5 consecutive days for 4 weeks

Table 1. Experimental groups and treatments.

2.6. Measurement of organ coefficients and the wet and dry weights of lung tissues

At the end of the treatment period, the animals were killed by arterial bloodletting. Their hearts, livers, spleens, kidneys, and other organs and tissues were then immediately removed and weighed, and the organ coefficient for each organ was calculated (organ coefficient = organ weight/body weight × 100%). The trachea and lungs were then removed and separated, and the lungs were stripped of their connective tissue. The connective tissues were soaked in water, and the wet lung weight (M) was measured. A 0.5 g lung tissue sample was then immersed in acetone for 3 days for degreasing and then cut into pieces, baked in an oven at 105°C for 12 h, and weighed to determine its dry weight (m). The dry weight of the lung was then calculated as 2 m×M.

2.7. Determination of total lung collagen (hydroxyproline)

Lung homogenates were prepared, and their hydroxyproline content was determined using the chloramine-T method, according to the instructions provided with the kit [27].

2.8. Counting and classification of cells in lung lavage fluid

The rats were killed by arterial bloodletting from the groin. The trachea was then removed, and a V-shaped opening was made at the 1/3 point of the lower trachea. One end of a small plastic hose was fitted with an eight-gauge needle, and the other end was inserted into the V-shaped opening and ligated to the lung using fixed lines. 5 mL of saline was taken up in a syringe, which was then affixed to the needle on the end of the tubing. The saline was slowly injected into the alveoli and then slowly withdrawn to yield approximately 3 mL of recovered liquid. The cells within this recovered liquid were counted and classified under a microscope.

2.9. Pathological analysis of lung tissues

First, the gross lung morphology was observed. The lung tissue was then fixed using formalin. Conventional paraffin sections were taken and stained with hematoxylin-eosin. The stained sections were then examined using an optical microscope (Olympus BX43). Lung tissue pathological changes and nodules pathological were graded, and stained lung tissue collagen fiber and reticular fiber hyperplasia were observed with Model BX43, Olympus Optical microscopy. The results obtained were evaluated according to the diagnostic criteria for pneumoconiosis specified in the national occupational health standards of the People"s Republic of China (GBZ25-2002).

2.10. Determination of the free silica contents of whole lung samples using the pyrophosphate method

Silica levels in lung samples were measured using the method for determining silica levels in dust samples described in Chinese national standard GBZ/T 192.4-2007 ("Determination of dust in the air of workplace—Part 4: Content of free silica in dust") [28]. Fresh rat lung samples were degreased, dried, and then crushed. Samples of the crushed material (0.10 g) were then analyzed using the above method.

3. Statistical analysis

All data were recorded in the form x ± s, where x is the mean value from a given number of observations and s is the associated standard deviation. The t-test was performed using the SPSS software package and used to analyze the significance of differences between groups, using a threshold value of $p < 0.05$.

4. Results

4.1. Clinical manifestations of silica exposure

In the period immediately following their injection with silica dust, the rats exhibited symptoms of dyspnea, did not eat much, and were sluggish. In the early stages of the treatment period, none of the silica-exposed groups exhibited any significant clinical abnormalities. In the later stages of the treatment period, individual rat weights decreased significantly. Four deaths occurred in total, one in the kombucha treatment group, one in the tetrandrine treatment group, one in the positive control group, and one in the negative control group. No deaths occurred in the Chinese herbal kombucha treatment group.

4.2. Changes in rat weight following silica exposure

The rats were weighed once per week during the treatment period. As can be seen in **Table 2**, there were no significant differences between the average weights for each group prior to their injection with silica. One week after exposure to the dust, the weight of the negative control group was significantly higher than that of the groups exposed to silica ($p < 0.01$). By the second week of the treatment period, the weights of the rats in the Chinese herbal kombucha and tetrandrine treatment groups were not significantly different to those of the negative control group. The weights of the rats in the kombucha treatment group and the positive control group also increased but remained significantly lower than those of the negative control animals ($p < 0.05$). This indicates that the Chinese herbal Kombucha and tetrandrine treatments both promoted the regaining of weight following silica exposure.

Treatment	10 days before silica exposure	2 days after treatment	9 days after treatment	16 days after treatment	23 days after treatment
Chinese herbal Kombucha	164.0 ± 7.1	202.8 ± 13.9ΔΔ	225.1 ± 18.9	240.1 ± 24.8	253.1 ± 29.3
Kombucha	163.6 ± 6.8	197.1 ± 11.2ΔΔ	222.4 ± 17.9Δ	238.1 ± 22.0	249.8 ± 29.0
Tetrandrine	164.87 ± 6.2	203.6 ± 12.8ΔΔ	231.7 ± 19.4	246.6 ± 30.0	259.4 ± 32.3
Positive control	165.6 ± 5.9	200.5 ± 12.6ΔΔ	220.8 ± 19.0Δ	237.2 ± 23.6	248.4 ± 26.7
Negative control	164.7 ± 6.6	217.7 ± 17.8	234.2 ± 23.8	248.7 ± 29.0	263.2 ± 31.1

ΔValue is significantly different to that for the negative control group ($p < 0.05$).

ΔΔ Value is significantly different to that for the negative control group ($p < 0.01$).

Table 2. Changes in the weight of dust-exposed rats over the course of the experimental period.

4.3. Organ coefficients after silica exposure

At the end of the treatment period, the hearts, livers, spleens, lungs, and kidneys of the rats in each group were removed and weighed, and the corresponding organ coefficients were calculated. The results (**Table 3**) indicate that there were no significant differences between the negative control group and any of the silica-exposed groups in terms of the organ coefficients for the liver, spleen, or kidney. However, the lung coefficients for all of the dust-exposed groups

http://dx.doi.org/10.5772/66970

were significantly greater ($p < 0.05$) than that for the negative control group. There were no significant differences between the lung coefficients for the various silica-exposed groups.

The lung coefficient data shown in **Table 3** demonstrate that the Chinese herbal kombucha and tetrandrine treatments inhibited the hyperblastosis of the lung tissue caused by silica exposure. **Table 3** also shows that the heart coefficient for the negative control group was significantly lower than those for the positive control group and the tetrandrine treatment group ($p < 0.05$). This suggests that both silica exposure and oral tetrandrine treatment have adverse effects on cardiac health.

Treatment	Heart	Liver	Spleen	Kidney	Lung
Chinese herbal Kombucha	$0.29 \pm 0.02^{*}$	3.35 ± 0.58	0.25 ± 0.03	0.68 ± 0.05	$1.82 \pm 0.80\Delta$
Kombucha	$0.28 \pm 0.03^{*}$	3.29 ± 0.59	0.25 ± 0.05	0.63 ± 0.05	$2.06 \pm 0.28\Delta$
Tetrandrine	$0.33 \pm 0.04\Delta$	3.64 ± 0.65	0.27 ± 0.05	0.68 ± 0.09	$1.46 \pm 0.52\Delta$
Positive control	$0.30 \pm 0.02^{*}\Delta$	3.16 ± 0.44	0.26 ± 0.04	0.64 ± 0.07	$1.96 \pm 0.38\Delta$
Negative control	$0.28 \pm 0.02^{*}$	3.34 ± 0.75	0.24 ± 0.05	0.66 ± 0.06	0.80 ± 0.19

* Value differs significantly from that for the tetrandrine treatment group ($p < 0.05$).

$^{\Delta}$ Value differs significantly from that for the negative control group (p.05).

Table 3. The influence of the various treatments on the organ coefficients of rats exposed to silica dust.

However, the heart coefficients for the kombucha and Chinese herbal kombucha treatment groups were significantly lower ($p < 0.05$) than that for the tetrandrine treatment group and were not significantly different from that for the negative control group. This indicates that kombucha and Chinese herbal kombucha are effective at mitigating the cardiotoxic effects of inhaling silica dust.

4.4. Cell counts in lung lavage fluid from silica-exposed rats

The negative control group had the lowest lung lavage fluid cell count (**Table 4**), averaging 0.308×10^9 cells/mL. Tetrandrine treatment yielded the highest average lavage fluid cell count ($7.20 \pm 13.62 \times 10^9$ cells/mL); one sample from this group had a count of 35×10^9 cells/mL. The cell counts in the lavage fluid from rats in other treatment groups were $2.46 \pm 1.78 \times 10^9$ cells/mL for the Chinese herbal kombucha group, $1.19 \pm 1.04 \times 10^9$ cells/mL for the kombucha group, and $1.12 \pm 0.75 \times 10^9$ cells/mL for the positive control group. Because of the considerable variation within each treatment group, there were no significant between-group differences.

In general, the greater the total number of cells within the lavage fluid, the more severe the case of silicosis. In conjunction with the finding that tetrandrine treatment suppresses hyperplasia in the lungs (**Table 3**), the high numbers of cells in the lung lavage fluid of the tetrandrine treatment group indicate that tetrandrine is a poor therapeutic agent due to its toxicity toward the tissues of the lung. The counted cells in the lung lavage fluid for each treatment group were sorted by type (**Table 4**). It was found that lymphocytes (L), neutral cells (N), giant divinatory cells (M) accounted for the vast majority of these cells.

Treatment	Total cells ($\times 10^9$/mL)	Cell type (%)		
		N	L	M
Positive control	1.12 ± 0.75	0.685 ± 0.004*	0.247 ± 0.067*	0.068 ± 0.0057*
Negative control	0.31 ± 0.19	0.272 ± 0.226	0.040 ± 0.051	0.692 ± 0.266
Chinese herbal Kombucha	2.46 ± 1.78	0.633 ± 0.320*	0.324 ± 0.290*	0.042 ± 0.034*
Kombucha	1.19 ± 1.04	0.718 ± 0.138*	0.256 ± 0.128*	0.027 ± 0.015*
Tetrandrine	7.20 ± 13.62	0.600 ± 0.192*	0.228 ± 0.244*	0.176 ± 0.210*

*: Value differs significantly from that for the negative control group ($p < 0.05$).

Table 4. The effects of the various treatments on the cell counts in lung lavage fluid from rats exposed to silica.

At the end of the treatment period, the most abundant cell type in the lavage fluid of the negative control group was M cells, followed by N and then L cells. Conversely, the lavage fluid of the dust-exposed groups was dominated by N cells, followed by L and then M cells. There were significant differences in the proportions of the different cell types between the negative control group and the silica-exposed groups ($p < 0.05$). M cells are phagocytes that are important for lung health. Their numbers are greatly reduced by dust exposure, causing the relative abundance of N cells to increase.

4.5. Hydroxyproline levels in the lungs of silica-exposed rats

Hydroxyproline assays were performed on lung samples taken from rats killed 1 week after the end of the treatment period (30 days after the onset of treatment) and from animals killed 3 weeks after the end of the treatment period (50 days after the onset of treatment). The results for the day 30 group are shown in **Table 5**. The only treatment group with hydroxyproline levels that were significantly different to those for the negative control group was that treated with non-Chinese herbal kombucha ($p < 0.05$). For the day 50 group, the hydroxyproline levels declined in the following order: positive control > kombucha treatment group > Chinese herbal kombucha treatment > tetrandrine treatment > negative control group. All of the silica-exposed groups other than

Treatment	Number of animals	Hydroxyproline level (mg/g*)	
		Day 30	Day 50
Chinese herbal Kombucha	6	0.45 ± 0.18	0.73 ± 0.22Δ
Kombucha	6	0.50 ± 0.14Δ	0.75 ± 0.12Δ
Tetrandrine	6	0.37 ± 0.09	0.56 ± 0.17
Positive control	6	0.45 ± 0.09	0.79 ± 0.28Δ
Negative control	6	0.34 ± 0.05	0.40 ± 0.06

*: Milligrams of hydroxyproline per gram of lung tissue.
Δ Value differs significantly from that for the negative control group ($p < 0.05$).

Table 5. The impact of the various treatments on hydroxyproline levels in the lungs of silica-exposed rats.

http://dx.doi.org/10.5772/66970

the tetrandrine treatment group had hydroxyproline levels that were significantly greater than that for the negative control group ($p < 0.05$). Since lung hydroxyproline levels are a biochemical indicator of pulmonary fibrosis, this suggests that tetrandrine is effective at inhibiting fibrosis.

In all cases, the hydroxyproline levels measured for the day 50 animals were substantially greater than those for the day 30 animals (**Table 5**). Moreover, the between-group differences for the day 50 animals were more significant than those for the day 30 animals. Both of these results indicate that lung fibrosis becomes more severe over time.

4.6. Lung pathology

Visual inspection of the pathological sections of the lungs of the experimental rats (**Figure 1A–E**) indicated that there were no abnormalities among the negative control group. However, signifi-

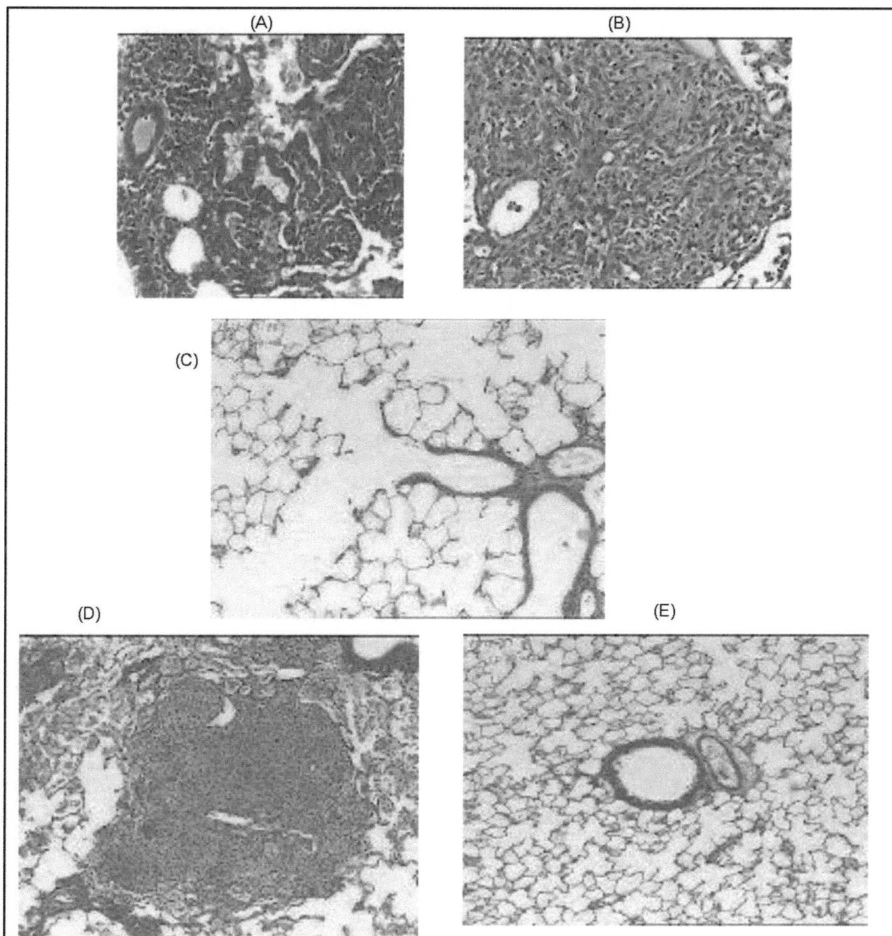

Figure 1. Pathological analysis of lung tissues from rats exposed to silica (400×). A: Chinese herbal kombucha treatment group; B: kombucha treatment group; C: tetrandrine treatment group; D: positive control group; E: negative control group.

cant partial lung consolidation was observed for the kombucha treatment group, the Chinese herbal kombucha treatment group, and the positive control group. The lesions in the sections taken from animals treated with non-Chinese herbal kombucha were particularly heavy, whereas the sections from animals treated with Chinese herbal kombucha were more similar to those for the positive control group. The sections from the tetrandrine treatment group exhibited less extensive lung consolidation and more evidence of lung inflammation.

4.7. Wet and dry lung weights

Among the experimental groups, the wet lung weight decreased in the following order: kombucha treatment group > positive control group > Chinese herbal kombucha treatment group > tetrandrine group > negative control group (**Table 6**). The difference between the values for the tetrandrine treatment group and the Chinese herbal Kombucha treatment group was not statistically significant, but that between the values for the positive control group and the tetrandrine group ($p < 0.05$). The dry lung weights for the various groups decreased in the same order as that for the wet lung weights. Based on these results, it was found that the water content of the lungs of rats treated with tetrandrine was relatively low (71.96 ± 0.74%) but that all other groups had similar lung water contents. This implies that tetrandrine treatment causes some level of tissue dehydration.

Treatment	Total wet lung weight (g)	Total dry lung weight (g)	Total lung moisture content (%)
Negative control	1.42 ± 0.43	0.34 ± 0.09	76.15 ± 1.31
Chinese herbal Kombucha	3.79 ± 0.93	0.90 ± 0.21	76.14 ± 1.10
Kombucha	4.78 ± 1.14	1.12 ± 0.18	76.19 ± 1.52
Tetrandrine	2.67 ± 0.26	0.75 ± 0.06	71.96 ± 0.74
Positive control	4.38 ± 0.85	1.04 ± 0.14	76.14 ± 1.63

Table 6. The effects of the tested treatments on wet and dry lung weight in silica-exposed rats.

Intrapulmonary levels of free silica were measured in lung samples from animals in each of the experimental groups. The highest free silica levels occurred in the tetrandrine treatment group (52.0 ± 12.0 mg). The value for the Chinese herbal kombucha group (38.0 ± 21.0) was significantly ($p < 0.05$) lower than that for both the tetrandrine group and the positive control group (44.0 ± 6.0 mg). Interestingly, the free silica level for the non-Chinese herbal kombucha treatment group was relatively high (54.0 ± 5.0 mg). These results suggest that treatment with Chinese herbal kombucha strongly promotes the discharge of free silica dust, whereas treatment with tetrandrine or non-Chinese herbal kombucha does not promote dust emission and may in fact cause some level of dust enrichment. Over the 30-day treatment period, the rate of silica discharge from the lungs of the rats treated with Chinese herbal kombucha was 0.47 ± 0.69 mg/day (**Table 7**).

http://dx.doi.org/10.5772/66970

Treatment	Whole lung free silica content (mg)	Free silica removed from the lung (mg)	Free silica clearance rate for the whole lung (%)	Silica discharge rate for the whole lung (mg/day)
Negative control	2.0 ± 1.0	–	–	–
Chinese herbal Kombucha	38.0 ± 21.0*	13.97 ± 20.65	27.92 ± 41.30	0.47 ± 0.69
Kombucha	54.0 ± 5.0	-2.46 ± 4.68	-4.92 ± 9.36	-0.08 ± 0.16
Tetrandrine	52.0 ± 12.0	-0.18 ± 11.78	-0.35 ± 23.55	-0.01 ± 0.39
Positive control	44.0 ± 6.0	5.81 ± 5.91	11.63 ± 11.83	0.25 ± 0.20

–: Because the rats in the negative control group were not exposed to silica, the analysis was not performed in this case.

*: Value differs significantly from that for the tetrandrine treatment group ($p < 0.05$).

Table 7. The effects of the tested treatments on dust removal from the lungs of silica-exposed rats.

5. Discussion

Silica dust is the main pathogenic factor of silicosis. Consequently, the development of effective methods for removing silica dust from the lungs will be essential for effectively treating this disease. This study explored the scope for using Chinese herbal and non-Chinese herbal kombucha preparations as dust-removing probiotic agents for treating silicosis and related conditions. At present, silicosis is treated using drugs such as oxypovidine, tetrandrine, and aluminum citrate, which only alleviate the symptoms of the disease; there is currently no cure. Tetrandrine is the most widely used drug for treating pneumoconiosis in China, and there is strong evidence that it directly or indirectly inhibits collagen gene transcription, thereby reducing collagen synthesis in the affected tissues. Long-term use of tetrandrine can reduce the severity of the respiratory symptoms of silicosis, and the number of lung infections suffered, as well as improving lung function. However, it can also cause skin discoloration and itching. Approximately 20% of all patients treated with tetrandrine experience sodium deficiency bloating, and approximately 9.8% experience impaired liver function [29, 30]. The results presented herein suggest that in addition to these effects, tetrandrine may be toxic to cardiac tissue and cause lung dehydration; the latter effect may be related to its known tendency to cause skin dehydration.

Our results indicate that tetrandrine treatment can suppress the formation of collagen in lung tissues. However, the cell counts in lung lavage fluid from tetrandrine-treated rats suggest that it has cytotoxic effects in the lungs and may inhibit the discharge of silica dust. This is consistent with the poor outcomes and severe side effects observed for patients that have been treated with tetrandrine for extended periods of time [29, 30]. As such, it may not be appropriate to use the inhibition of collagen synthesis in lung tissue as the main indicator of effectiveness when evaluating the performance of drugs for the treatment of silicosis.

Aside from medication, the most common treatment for pneumoconiosis-type diseases such as silicosis is large-volume whole-lung lavage. This method involves repeatedly flushing the lungs with saline under intravenous anesthesia, together with mechanical ventilation, to remove the pathogenic factor [31]. However, there are several groups of patients that are not suitable for large-volume whole-lung lavage, including those with (1) conditions that affect blood clotting; (2) severe tracheal or bronchial deformities; (3) illnesses or dysfunctions of the heart, brain, liver, kidneys, or other major organs; (4) cancers or compromised immune systems; (5) active tuberculosis; (6) pulmonary bullae, especially subpleural bullae greater than 2 cm in diameter; (7) severely low pulmonary function; and (8) severe emphysema or related conditions [31]. An analysis of 5000 cases in which large-volume whole-lung lavage was performed to treat pneumoconiosis or some other lung disorders indicated that the short-term effects (1–3 years) of the treatment are good, but its long-term effects (6–7 years) are not significant. In most cases, lavage causes reductions in chest tightness (reported by 99% of patients), chest pain (reported by 86% of all patients), and shortness of breath (reported by 88% of all patients), with these beneficial effects lasting for around 3 years. The average amount of dust cleared from each lung was 3000 to 5000 mg, including 70–200 mg of free silica. However, extensive removal of pulmonary alveolar macrophages was also observed [32]. While some of the dust and other foreign material are removed from the lungs by lavage, the process can cause significant secondary damage, resulting in complications such as tuberculosis. Additionally, lung lavage is expensive, and much of the cost is borne by the patient; since most pneumoconiosis patients have economic difficulties, it would be desirable to find a less costly alternative.

Our experiments using silica-exposed rats demonstrated that spraying with Chinese herbal kombucha preparations has no toxic side effects and effectively promotes the discharge of silica dust from the lungs. The silica dust exhaust rate for rats (average body weight: 0.200 kg) treated with Chinese herbal Kombucha was 0.4 mg/day. Simple linear extrapolation suggests that if a human with a body weight of 65 kg were subjected to the same treatment, the corresponding rate of silica removal would be 130 mg/day. Rats passively accept the aerosol therapy during the test, but a human undergoing treatment would actively inhale the Chinese herbal probiotic. It is therefore possible that the results achieved in clinical trials might be even better than those observed with the rat model.

The average amount of dust cleared from each lung during lavage is 3000–5000 mg. Based on the results obtained in this work, it would require 23–38 days of spraying with Chinese herbal kombucha to achieve a similar effect. This is consistent with the results obtained when a single pneumoconiosis patient was treated by spraying with Chinese herbal kombucha for 3 months (see the case report presented in Appendix 1). The patient experienced significant reductions in the severity of his symptoms within a month, and X-rays taken at the end of the treatment period demonstrated that the treatment had significant beneficial effects on his pulmonary health. Because Chinese herbal kombucha preparations have no toxic side effects and can be also used to treat TB patients and those with cardiopulmonary dysfunctions, they could potentially replace lung lavage as a treatment for pneumoconiosis.

It has been demonstrated that the amount of dust in the lungs of pneumoconiosis sufferers ranges from 0 to 60 g. Based on the system used to classify cases of pneumoconiosis, first-stage cases occur when the lungs contain 0–15 g of dust; this causes dust reticulocyte fibrosis. Second-stage cases (15–30 g dust) are characterized by the appearance of mixed nodules due to reticulocyte fibrosis. Third-stage cases (30–60 g of dust) are characterized by the appearance of converged fibrosis nodules [33]. Given a dust discharge rate of 130 mg/day, 115 days of treatment with Chinese herbal kombucha would be required to discharge the bulk of the dust in first-stage cases, 231 days would be required to treat second-stage cases, and 461 days of treatment would be required for third-stage cases. A treatment cycle of around 1 year should thus be sufficient to treat patients with stage I or II pneumoconiosis. However, the lung X-rays in the single-patient case study (see Appendix 1) showed that significant quantities of dust were still present within the lungs after 3 months of treatment, so 2–3 treatment cycles may be required for the complete removal of dust from the lungs in some cases. Even if the treatment only removed dust from the surface tissues of the pulmonary alveolae, significant improvements in lung function would be achieved. However, longer treatment periods may be required to clear deep-seated dust from the lungs.

In this work, two probiotic mixtures were used to treat silicosis. Interestingly, only the Chinese herbal kombucha preparations had unambiguously beneficial effects on dust emission. Non-Chinese herbal kombucha did not promote dust emission, so it appears that the combination of Chinese herbal extracts and the kombucha culture has advantageous synergistic effects. The plant species used to prepare the Chinese herbal kombucha are known to have antitussive, expectorant, and antiasthma function, as well as protecting against respiratory pathogens. Based on these results, they also seem to promote the health of pulmonary tissues and dust emission mediated by the cilia. Kombucha cultures contain two groups of symbiotic microbes: xylinum and yeasts. Xylinum generates bacterial cellulose from the ethanol produced by the yeast; bacterial cellulose is an efficient adsorbing agent that will adhere to dust particles and other substances, thereby facilitating their removal via expectoration.

It should be noted that the treatments examined in this work were only applied over a period of 1 month. This is relatively short, and it would be desirable to study the effects of treatment with Chinese herbal kombucha over a longer period of time. In addition, the composition of the Chinese herbal kombucha mixture has not been optimized to maximize its therapeutic effect, and it is likely that more extensive research in this area would result in the identification of more potent mixtures. Finally, it would be desirable to determine the precise mechanisms by which treatment with Chinese herbal kombucha promotes the removal of dust from the lungs. Overall, however, the results presented in this work represent the first effective use of an Chinese herbal probiotic to promote the emission of dust from the lungs and the alleviation of inflammation in cases of silicosis. This could have significant consequences for the treatment of silicosis and other pneumoconiosis diseases, and more generally for treating conditions involving inflammation of the lungs such as lung protein deposition psychosis. It is very easy to produce and use the Chinese herbal Kombucha. Therefore, the Chinese herbal

Kombucha would help to globally remove silicosis, pneumoconiosis, and similar diseases in the future.

Acknowledgements

This research was supported in part by earmarked funds from the China Agriculture Research System (CARS-32-hnjsj) and the basic scientific fund of the Tropical Crops Genetic Resources Institute at the Chinese Academy of Tropical Agriculture Science (009).

Appendix 1

A case of gold pneumoconiosis and tuberculosis treated by spraying with Chinese herbal Kombucha

In 2011, I was informed that my brother-in-law had been diagnosed with pneumoconiosis and tuberculosis, presenting with a cough and serious dyspnea. At the time, he was not able to work. Given the lack of success, he had experienced with existing treatments, and after deep and long consideration, I suggested that the Chinese herbal kombucha inhalation as a way of treating his pneumoconiosis. Kombucha contains two symbiotic microorganisms: xylinum and yeast [34]. Xylinum secretes bacterial cellulose from the eyelets of its cell walls. Bacterial cellulose is very effective at adsorbing heavy metal ions and various toxic organic compounds [35]. I therefore hypothesized that if kombucha was administered into the patient's lung, mineral dust and proteinaceous material in the lung would be adsorbed on the cellulose and could then be discharged by expectoration. To further enhance the potentially beneficial effects of the kombucha preparation, it was made using aqueous extracts of health-promoting Chinese herbs (licorice, luohanguo, and chrysanthemum) to yield a substance known as Chinese herbal kombucha. This preparation had previously proven very effective at removing silica dust from the lungs in a rat model of silicosis. The patient was instructed to spray the Chinese herbal kombucha mixture into his mouth and nose on a daily basis from 2012-2-21 to 2012-5-21, over a period of 3 months. At the end of this period, the patient reported significant reductions in chest tightness, coughing, and other symptoms and was able to return to work. X-ray images of the patient's chest were acquired before the commencement of the treatment and after its conclusion (see **Figure 2**). The treatment reduced the absorption and shadowing caused by lung nodules, made the hilar slightly smaller, and resulted in somewhat less opaque images than those acquired prior to the initiation of treatment. Importantly, the contrast in the non-affected lung tissues was identical in both sets of X-ray images, suggesting that the apparent beneficial effects of Chinese kombucha inhalation. While the X-rays suggest that only a small proportion of the total mineral dust within the patient's lungs was removed, this was apparently sufficient to reestablish effective oxygenation and ventilation, significantly improving lung function. Given that these results were achieved with a relatively short treatment period, it seems reasonable to suggest that more mineral dust might have been removed if the treatment had been extended.

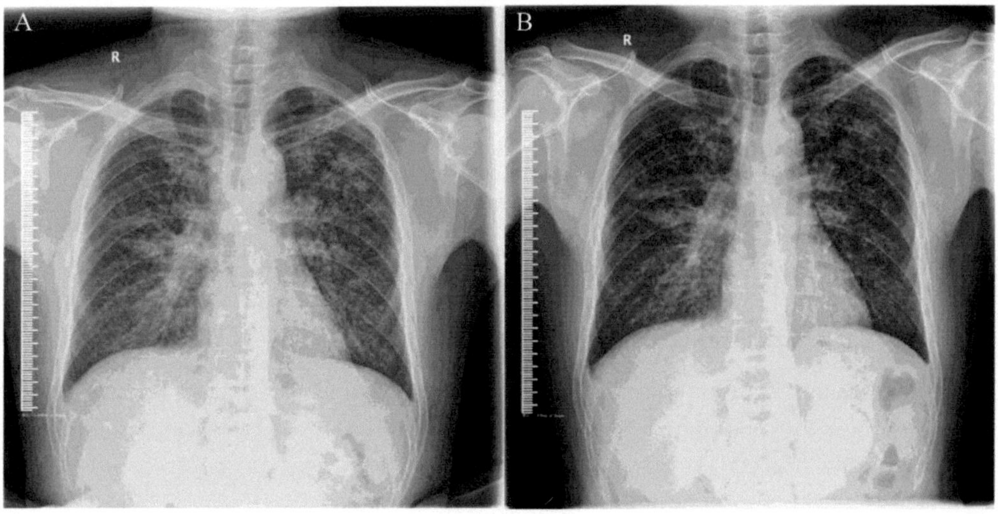

Figure 2. A gold pneumoconiosis patient treated by spraying with Chinese herbal kombucha. A: X-ray taken before treatment. B: X-ray taken after the conclusion of the treatment period.

Pneumoconiosis is a serious occupational disease caused by inhaling fine mineral dust. Recent reports indicate that more than 37.7 million workers have been exposed to crystalline silica dust in China, India, the USA, and Europe [36]. Pneumoconiosis has long been regarded as an incurable disease, and no significant breakthroughs in its treatment have been made during the last decade [37]. The only known effective treatment is whole-lung lavage, which involves washing out mineral dust and other foreign substances from the lungs. However, it is an expensive and painful surgical procedure that cannot be applied to many patients and has a range of potentially adverse consequences. Moreover, it has no beneficial effects in the long term. On average, whole-lung lavage removes 6–10 g of mineral dust from the patient's lungs [38]. In experiments using a rat silicosis model, treatment with Chinese herbal kombucha resulted in a silica excretion rate of 0.47 mg/day from the lungs. Given that the average bodyweight of the rats in the experiment was 0.2 kg and assuming a body weight of 65 kg for humans, simple linear extrapolation suggests that if the same treatment was applied in humans, the resulting rate of silica/mineral dust excretion would be 152.75 mg/day. Thus, treatment with Chinese herbal kombucha treatment for 40–65 days should achieve approximately the same level of mineral discharge as can be achieved in a single session of lung lavage. However, the rats would have passively inhaled the kombucha, whereas a human patient would presumably actively inhale it. As such, it is possible that the rate of removal may be greater in human patients. Chinese herbal kombucha inhalation is much less costly than existing methods for treating pneumoconiosis. Together with the promising preliminary results reported herein and those obtained using the rat model, it may be a useful alternative to whole-lung lavage and other more invasive medical procedures for the treatment of pneumoconiosis and other lung disorders.

Author details

Sheng-jun Jiang[1, 2*], Nai-fang Fu[1], Zhi-chao Dong[1], Chang-hui Luo[1], Jun-cai Wu[1], Yan-yan Zheng[3], Yong-jin Gan[3], Jian-an Ling[3], Heng-qiu Liang[3], Dan-yu Liang[3], Jing Xie[3], Xiao-qin Chen[3], Xian-jun Li[3], Rui-hui Pan[3], Zuo-Xing Chen[3] and Lu-lu Zhang[4]

*Address all correspondence to: 18708938111@139.com

1 Tropical Crop Genetic Resources Institute, Tropical Academy of Tropical Agriculture Science, Hainan, China

2 Hainan Mulada Biosci & Biotech corperation, Haikou city, Hainan, China

3 Guangxi Zhuang Autonomous Region Institute for Chemical Toxicity Testing, Guangxi Zhuang Autonomous Region Academy for the Prevention and Treatment of Occupational Disease, Guangxi, China

4 Nongken Sanya Hospital in Hainan Province, Sanya, China

References

[1] Costantini LM, Gilberti RM, Knecht DA. The Phagocytosis and Toxicity of Amorphous Silica. *PLoS One* 2011; 6(2): e14647.

[2] Chen W, Liu Y, Wang H, Hnizdo E, Sun Y, Su L, et al. Long-term exposure to silica dust and risk of total and cause-specific mortality in workers: a cohort study. *PLoS Med* 2012; 9(4): e1001206.

[3] Ministry of Health of the People's Republic of China. Annual health statistical report in 2009. Beijing: Ministry of Health of the People's Republic of China. 2009.

[4] World Health Organization Global Occupational Health Network. Elimination of silicosis. Gohnet Newsletter 12. Geneva: World Health Organization Global Occupational Health Network. 2007.

[5] US National Institute for Occupational Safety and Health. Health effects of occupational exposure to respirable crystalline silica. Washington District of Columbia: US Department of Health and Human Services. 2002.

[6] Kauppinen T, Toikkanen J, Pedersen D, Young R, Ahrens W, Boffetta P, et al. Occupational exposure to carcinogens in the European Union. *Occup Environ Med* 2000; 57: 10–18.

[7] Greenwalt CJ, Steinkraus KH, Ledford RA. Kombucha, the fermented tea: microbiology, composition, and claimed health effects. *J Food Prot* 2000; 63: 976–981.

[8] Ross P, Mayer R, Benziman M. Cellulose biosynthesis and function in bacteria. *Microbiol Rev* 1991; 55(1): 35–58.

[9] Tang SJ, Yang XX, Hong F. Production of bacterial cellulose by Kombucha. *J Cellulose Sci Tech* 2012; 20: 40–45.

[10] Zhu CL, Li F, You QS. Preparation of nanometer biomaterial bacterial cellulose and observation of its ultra-structure. *J Biomed Eng Res* 2008; 27: 287–290.

[11] Argun ME, Dursun S, Ozdemir C, Karatas M. Heavy metal adsorption by modified oak sawdust: thermodynamics and kinetics. *J Hazard Mater* 2007; 141: 77–85.

[12] Chen S, Zou Y, Yan Z, Shen W, Shi S, Zhang X, et al. Carboxymethylated-bacterial cellulose for copper and lead ion removal. *J Hazard Mater* 2009; 161: 1355–1359.

[13] T, Kondo k, Ohto K, Inoue k, Baba Y. Preparation of phosphorylated bacterial cellulose as an adsorbent for metal ions. *React Funct Polym* 2008; 68: 376–383.

[14] Lu M, Guan XH. Adsorption mechanism of bacterial cellulose to heavy metal ions. *Chem Eng* 2012; 40: 29–33.

[15] Zhou H, Sun DP, Zhu CL, Xu CY. Study on the adsorption of noxious substances in human body by bacterial cellulose. *J Cellulose Sci Tech* 2009; 17: 41–46.

[16] Wang YQ, Zhang QS. Study on the absorption property for formaldehyde by bacterial cellulose. *Jiangsu Constr* 2011; 3: 67–70.

[17] Zhang MF, Shen YQ. Effects of licorice and its extracts on respiratory system. *Drugs Clinic* 2010; 25: 262–267.

[18] Menegazzi M, Di Paola R, Mazzon E, Genovese T, Crisafulli C, Dal Bosco M, et al. Glycyrrhizin attenuates the development of carrageenan-induced lung injury in mice. *Pharmacol Res* 2008; 58: 22–31.

[19] Chen Y, Jia EL. The research progress of the chemical constituents and pharmacological action of Momordica grosvenori. *Pharmaceutical J PLA* 2011; 27: 171–174.

[20] Li J, Li PB, Yuan GJ. The antitussive effect of water extrat of grosvenor momordica fruit. *J Hainan Medical College* 2008; 14: 16–18.

[21] Rajic A, Akihisa T. Inhibition of trypsin and chymotrypsin by anti-inflammatory triterpenoids from Compositae flowers. *Planta Med* 2001; 67: 599–604.

[22] Shen CL, Yeh JK, Cao JJ, Tatum OL, Dagda RY, Wang JS. Synergistic effects of green tea polyphenols and alphacalcidol on chronic inflammation-induced bone loss in female rats. *Osteoporos Int* 2010; 21: 1841–1852.

[23] Lu A,Yin J, Hu X, Zhang P, Hu B. A Study on morphology of tea fungus and inhibition effect of its culture fluid. *J Xuzhou Normal Uni* 2004; 22: 73–75.

[24] Xie QM, Tang HF, Chen JQ, Bian RL. Pharmacological actions of tetrandrine in inflammatory pulmonary diseases. *Acta Pharmacol Sin* 2002; 23: 1107–1113.

[25] Faxuan W, Qin Z, Dinglun Z, Tao Z, Xiaohui R, Liqiang Z, et al. Altered microRNAs expression profiling in experimental silicosis rats. *J Toxicol Sci* 2012; 37: 1207–1215.

[26] Gao HS, Rong Xue, Peng Ding, Chen NF, Bing Meng, Zhao HB, et al. Cross-talk of the related bioactivity mediators in serum after injection of soluble TNF-α receptor on silicosis model of rats. *Toxicol Ind Health* 2011; 27: 607–616.

[27] Wang X, Chen Y, Lv L, Chen J. Silencing CD36 gene expression results in the inhibition of latent-TGF-beta1 activation and suppression of silica-induced lung fibrosis in the rat. *Respir Res* 2009; 10: 36.

[28] Wang XT, Liu J, Liu LH, Zhao JY. Analysis of influencing factors on infrared spectroscopic determination of the content of free silica in quartz sand. *Zhonghua Lao Dong Wei Sheng Zhi Ye Bing Za Zhi* 2011; 29: 622–625.

[29] He YX, Miu Q, Liu BC. Effects of polyvinylpyridine oxide on gene expression of type I and III collagens in experimental silicosis. *J Pharmaceutical* 1995; 30: 271–273.

[30] Chen ZP, Su WG, Yan S. Therapeutic effect of tetrandrine on patients with pneumoconiosis. *J Clin Pulmonary Med* 2012; 17: 1226–1227.

[31] Gao J, Zhang Z, Ji X, Cao X, Xiao X, Hu X, et al. Further discussion on the indications and contraindications in whole-lung lavage. *Occup Health* 2011; 27: 410–412.

[32] Zhang ZH, Liu H, Ma GX. Clinical analysis of the 5000 cases of pneumoconiosis and other lung disorders treated by large volume whole lung lavage treatment. *J Conval Med* 2009; 10: 956–960.

[33] Zhang QF, Zhang Z, Mao GG, zhang Q, Du Y. Data analysis and experimental study on pathogenic therapy or lung lavage for dust removal. *Occup Med* 2000; 27: 4–6.

[34] Greenwalt C J, Steinkraus K H, Ledford R A. Kombucha, the fermented tea: microbiology, composition, and claimed health effects. *J Food Prot* 2000; 63: 976–981.

[35] Chen S, Zou Y, Yan Z, et a1. Carboxymethylated-bacterial cellulose for copper and lead ion removal. *J Hazard Mater* 2009; 161: 1355–1359.

[36] Chen W, Liu Y, Wang H,et al. Long-term exposure to silica dust and risk of total and cause-specific mortality in Chinese workers: a cohort study. *PLoS Med* 2012; 9: e1001206.

[37] Centers for Disease Control and Prevention (CDC). Silicosis-related years of potential life lost before age 65 years—nited States, 1968–2005. *MMWR Morb Mortal Wkly Rep* 2008; 57: 771–775.

[38] Zhang Z, Liu H, Ma G, et al. Clinical analysis of 5000 cases of large volume whole lung lavage treatment of pneumoconiosis and other lung disorders. *Chin J Convalescent Med* 2009; 10: 956–960 (in Chinese)